DISCOVER YOUR SMILE AND HIDE YOUR BRACES

THE TRUTH ABOUT CLEAR TOOTH ALIGNERS

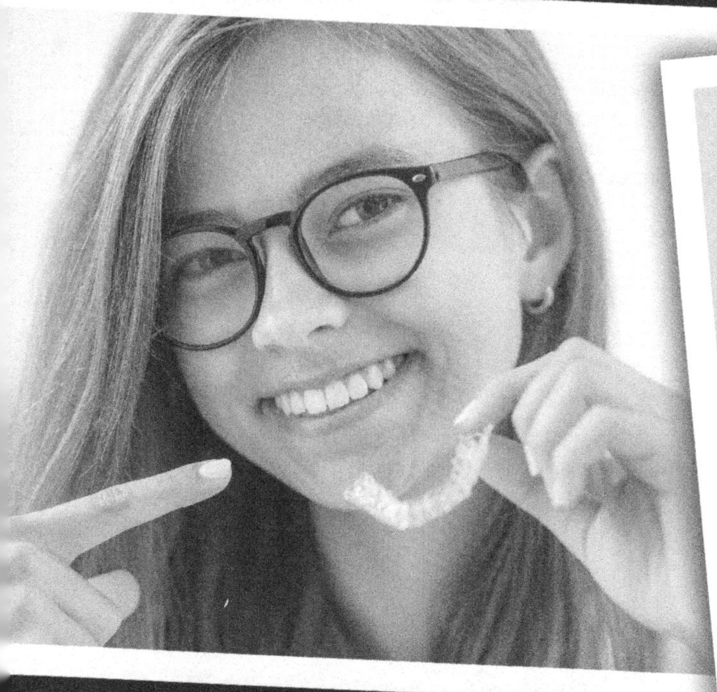

TIMOTHY C. SCANLAN, DDS, MS

Printed in the United States of America.

10 9 8 7 6 5 4 3 2 1

ISBN: 978-1-970095-12-8

Cover design by Art in Motion Graphic Design LLC
Layout design by Art in Motion Graphic Design LLC

TABLE OF CONTENTS

Chapter 1: What is Invisalign®?

The History of Invisalign 7

Invisalign Overview 13

Treatment for Teens 18

5 Reasons to Consider Invisalign for Your Teen 24

Information for Parents 30

Treatment for Adults 41

5 Reasons to Consider Invisalign as an Adult 48

Chapter 2: How Invisalign Works

How Your Treatment Plan is Developed 57

How Your Aligners are Created 59

Receiving Your First Aligners 60

Living with Clear Aligners 61

TABLE OF CONTENTS (continued)

Your Treatment Timeline 65

Post Treatment Care 67

Chapter 3: Treatment Comparisons

Which Type of Invisalign is Right for Me? 72

Questions to Ask Yourself About Invisalign 79

Differences Between Invisalign and Mail Order Aligners 84

Treatment Comparison Chart 92

Chapter 4: Cases that Invisalign Corrects

Crowded or Crooked Teeth 95

Overbite 98

Underbite 102

Crossbite 106

TABLE OF CONTENTS (continued)

Gap Teeth 110

Open Bite 115

General Teeth Straightening 119

Chapter 5: The Cost of Invisalign

Ways to Pay for Invisalign Treatment 123

Chapter 6: What About Wisdom Teeth?

Some Advice on Wisdom Teeth: Keeping it Straight 130

Chapter 7: Taking the Next Step

Getting Started 138

Your Personal Smile Assessment 141

About the Author 147

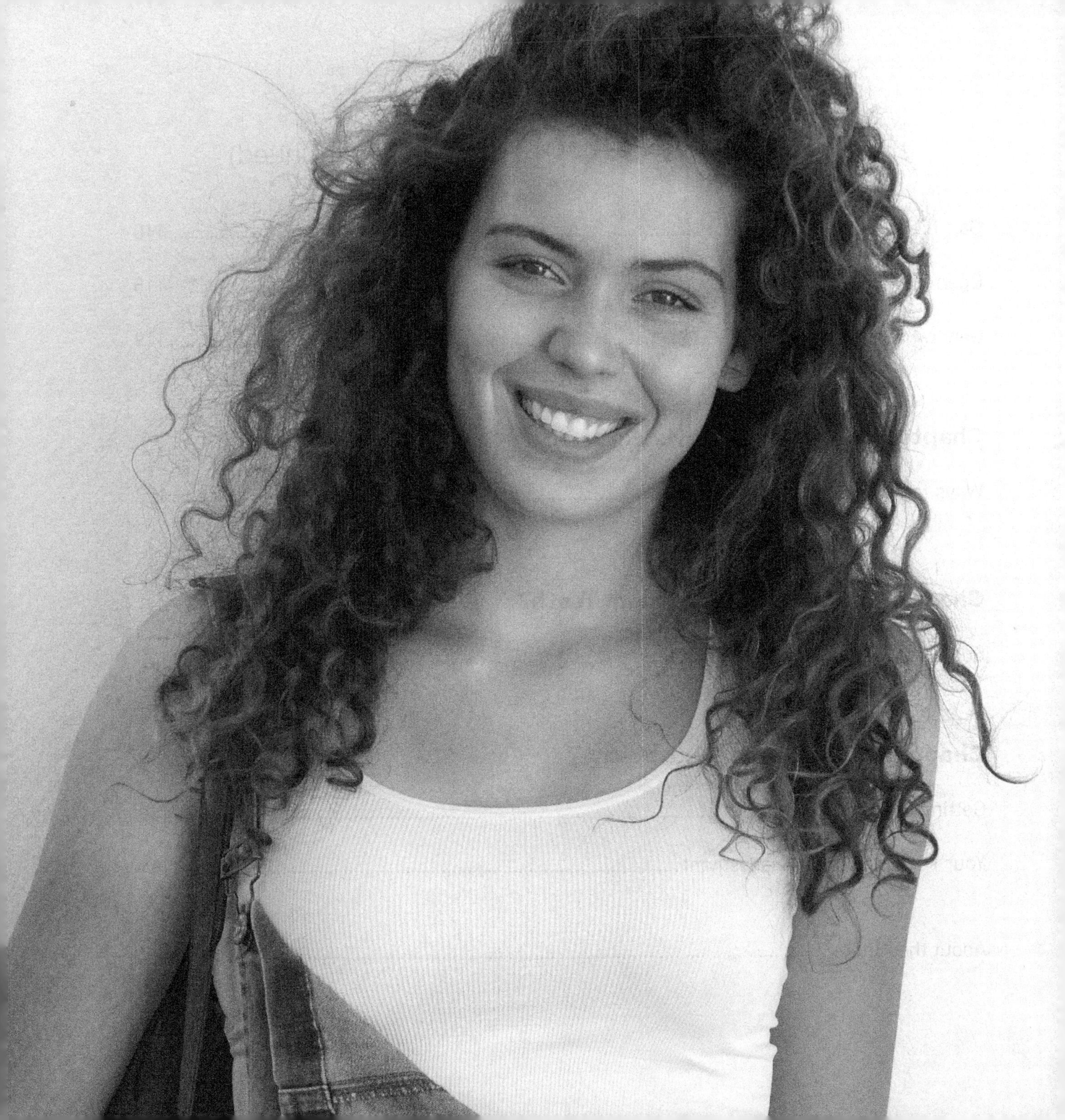

Chapter 1: What is Invisalign?

Invisalign is a highly effective method of straightening teeth that has become one of the most popular types of braces in recent years. It offers many advantages over traditional, metal braces, such as eliminating wires and brackets, but one of the largest benefits of Invisalign is that the aligners are completely clear and almost invisible to the naked eye. This allows a patient to show off a beautiful smile even during the process of straightening their teeth, which no doubt is one of the reasons why more and more patients are choosing this method as a way of achieving the smile of their dreams.

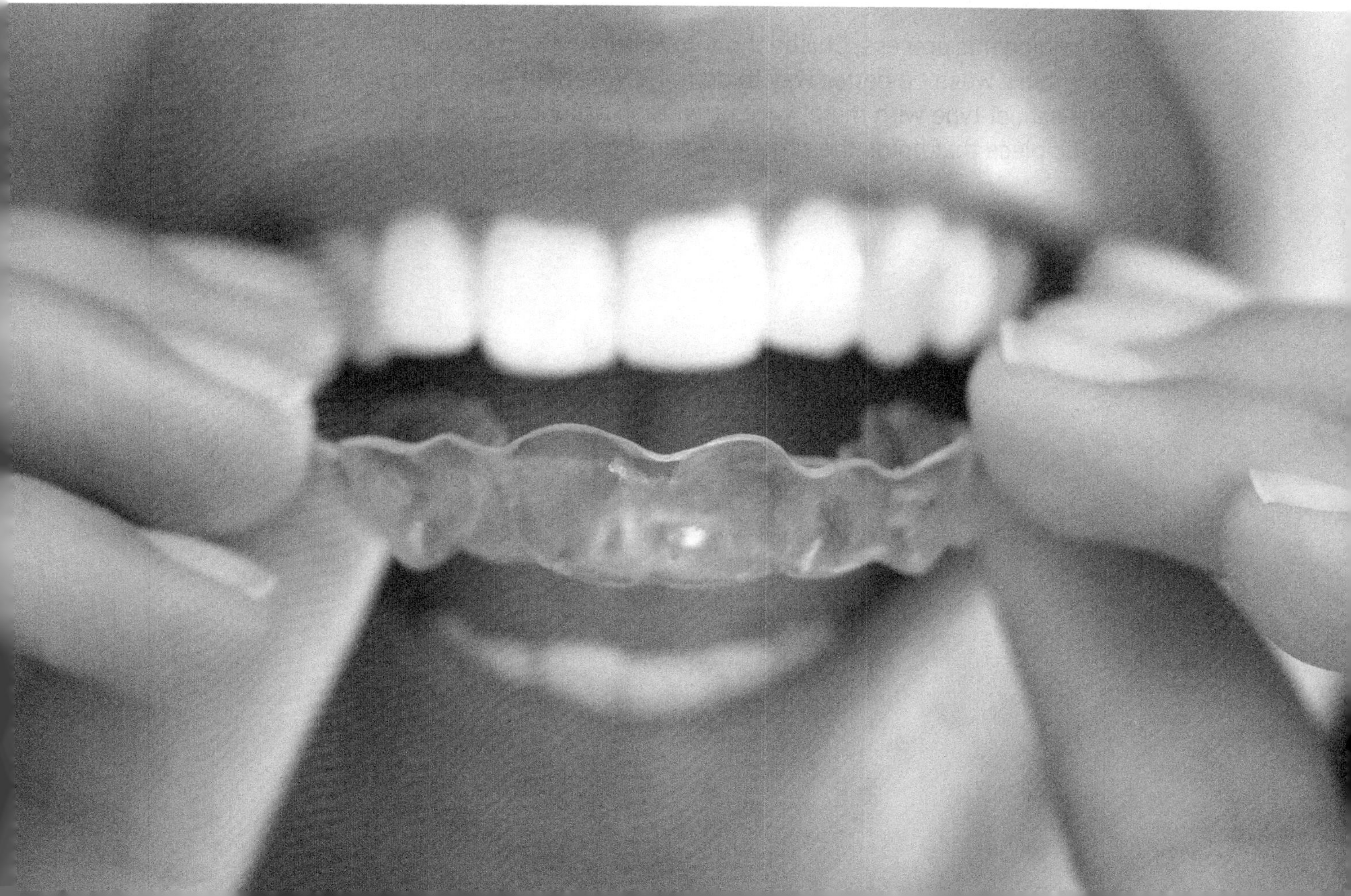

The History of Invisalign

Did you know that the person who invented Invisalign was actually a patient and *not a doctor?*

In the late 1990s, a young student at Stanford named Zia Chishti was finishing up orthodontic treatment which he underwent in order to correct an issue with crowded teeth. Anyone who has worn traditional metal braces can attest to the fact that getting your braces taken off is a laborious and time consuming process - and there are many steps, including making molds of your teeth. Braces are also adhered to your teeth with a special glue, and it can sometimes take multiple cleanings for your doctor to fully remove it from your teeth.

While undergoing this process, Chishti thought about how cumbersome this process was, and he wondered if there wasn't a better way to do it. He was then given a retainer - which at the time was the old-school type with metal wires that loop around the teeth to hold them in alignment with a plastic piece that holds the retainer against the roof of your mouth.

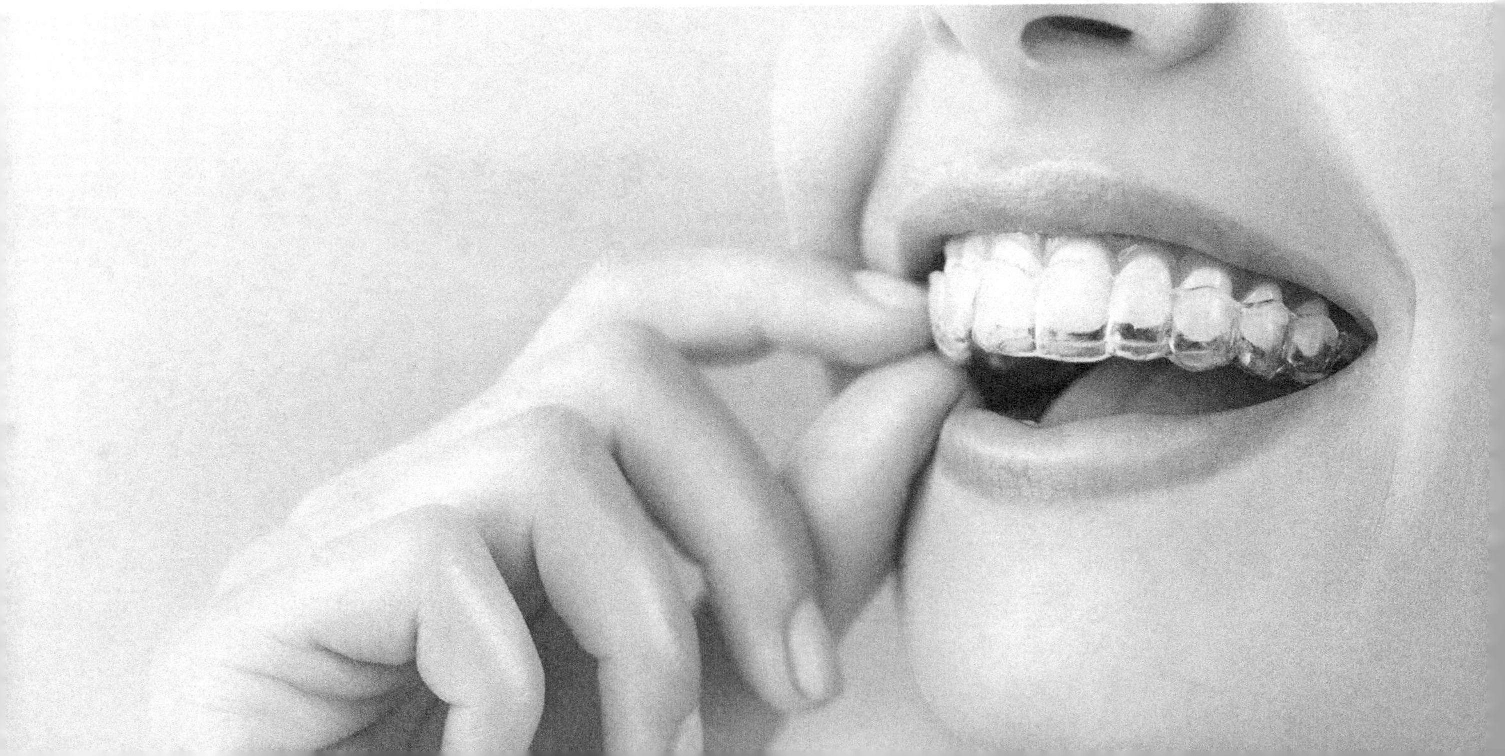

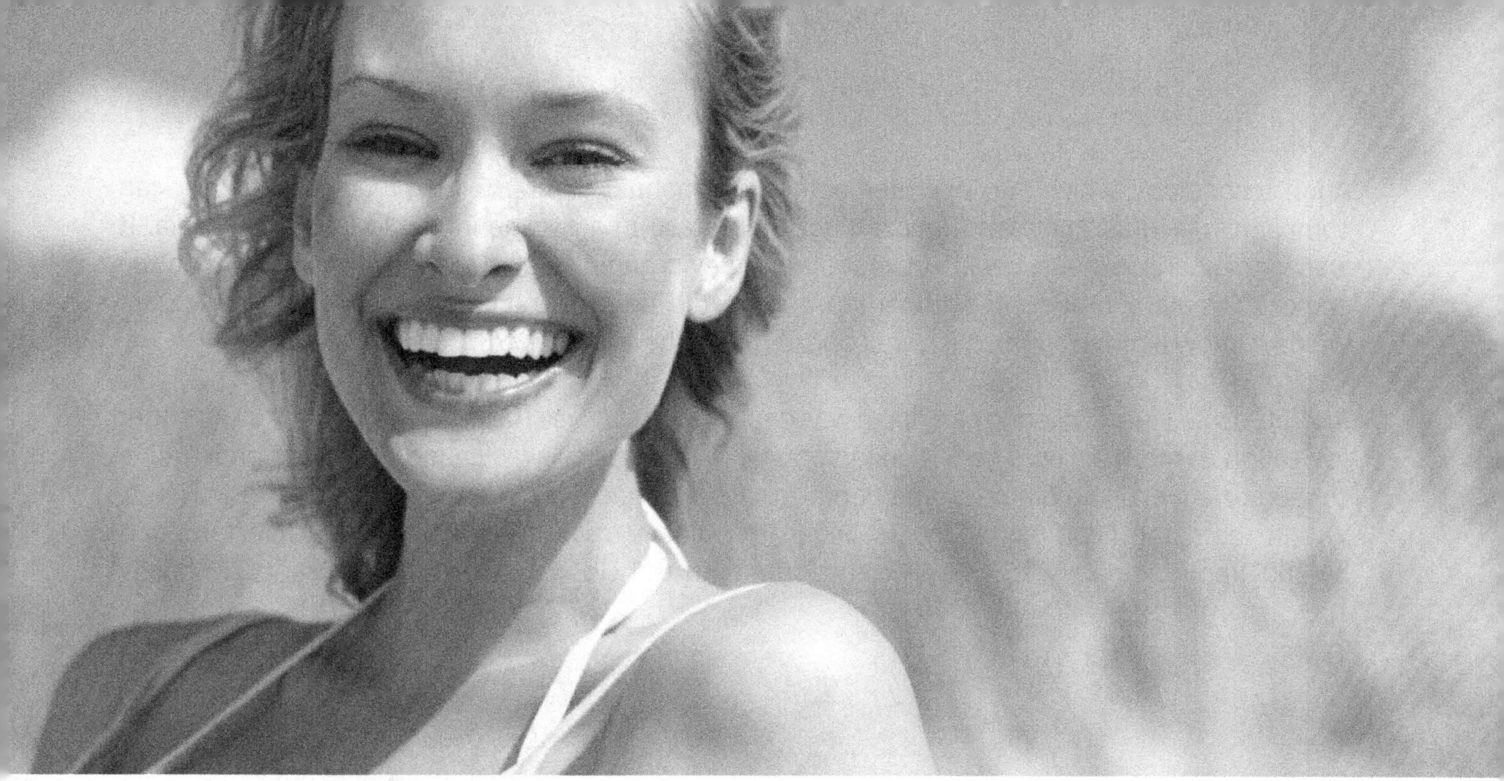

In examining this retainer, he realized that if this device could keep the teeth that braces had fixed in place, then there might be a way to create a similar device that would take care of the entire straightening process. This would have far more benefits that metal braces, and it would eliminate the tedious process he had just went through when his braces were removed.

Another thing that Chishti learned about having braces was that they were very inconvenient, especially as an adult patient. While it was routine for teenagers to have them, being an adult with braces was a source of looks from strangers and other stigma. This further motivated him to continue his idea to come up with a way that the process of straightening teeth could be easier and less invasive.

He discussed his idea with fellow Stanford University Kelsey Wirth, and the two teamed up and began exploring ways they could make his idea a reality. Using Chishti's experience with orthodontics and their business acumen as MBA students, they conducted research for over a year, ultimately bringing on two additional partners. In 1997, they formed a business called

Align Technology, which they operated at first in a manner similar to how many great American companies such as Apple and Amazon got their start: in a garage in Menlo Park, California. It was in this garage that, a couple of years later, they created a set of aligners which could do the same job as metal braces but with far less hassle, discomfort, and time investment - the product we now know as Invisalign which was approved by the FDA in 1998.

In 2000, a massive marketing campaign was deployed which was the movement that truly brought Invisalign to the masses. The $31 million dollar TV campaign was called the "most aggressive consumer advertising plan that the dental profession has ever seen," by the New York Times. Within the same year, orthodontists began to receive training in the Invisalign system, and by 2001, approximately 75% of all orthodontists in the US were Invisalign providers. Shortly

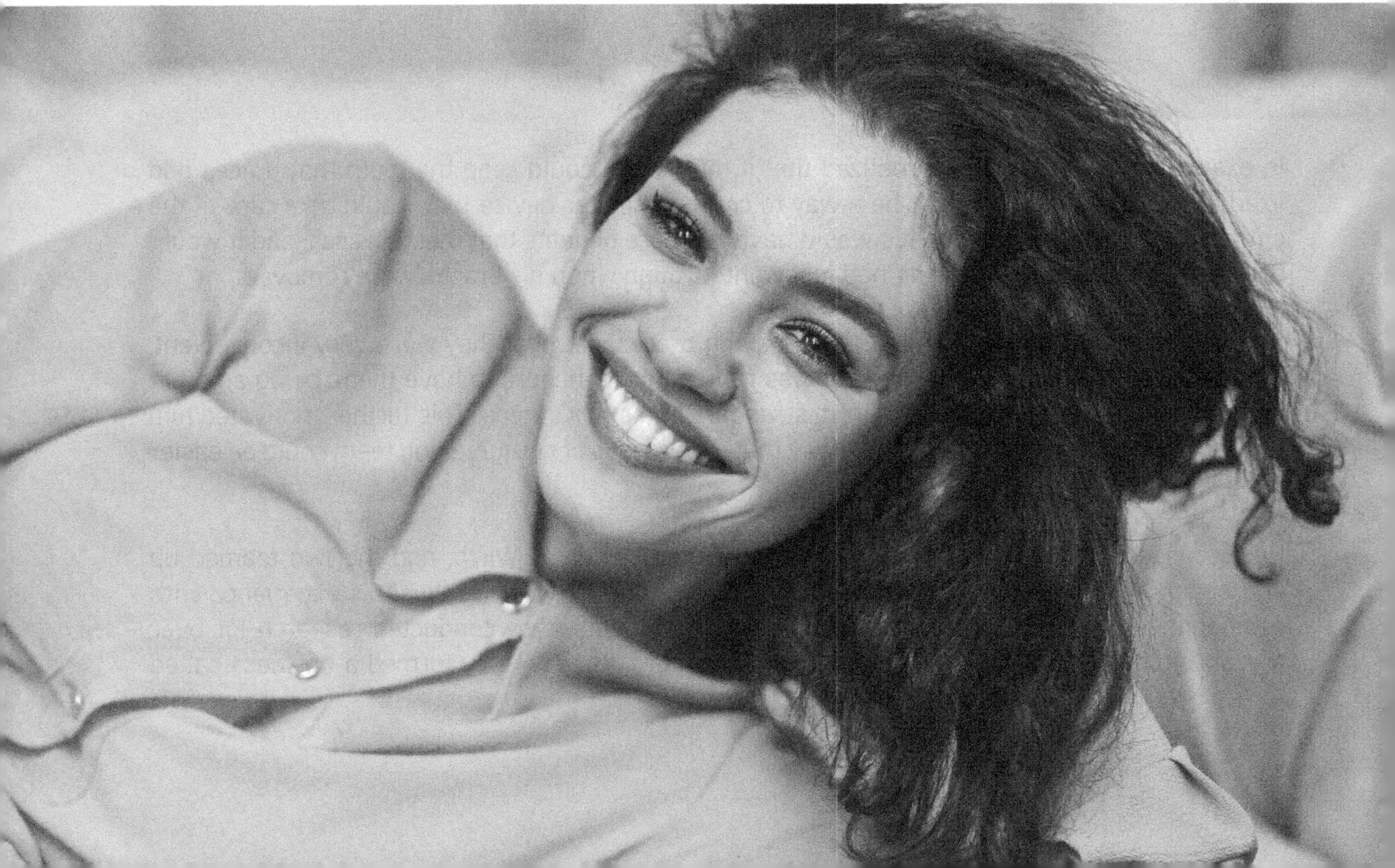

after, the company also offered the opportunity for general dentists to also offer this system of treatment to their patients. The rest, as they say, is history.
From the start, Align Technology's focus was to help bring better dental solutions for both doctors and patients and to make those solutions not just effective, but affordable. Today the publicly traded company has over 3,000 world wide employees and they have continued their dedication to improving lives with great smiles by innovating new products and systems that make a great product even better.

As of this writing, Invisalign has been used in more than 90 countries and has successfully straightened teeth for more than 5 million people worldwide. With a proven track record of success and technology that is always improving, it's easy to see why it is recommended by so many dental professionals including our office.

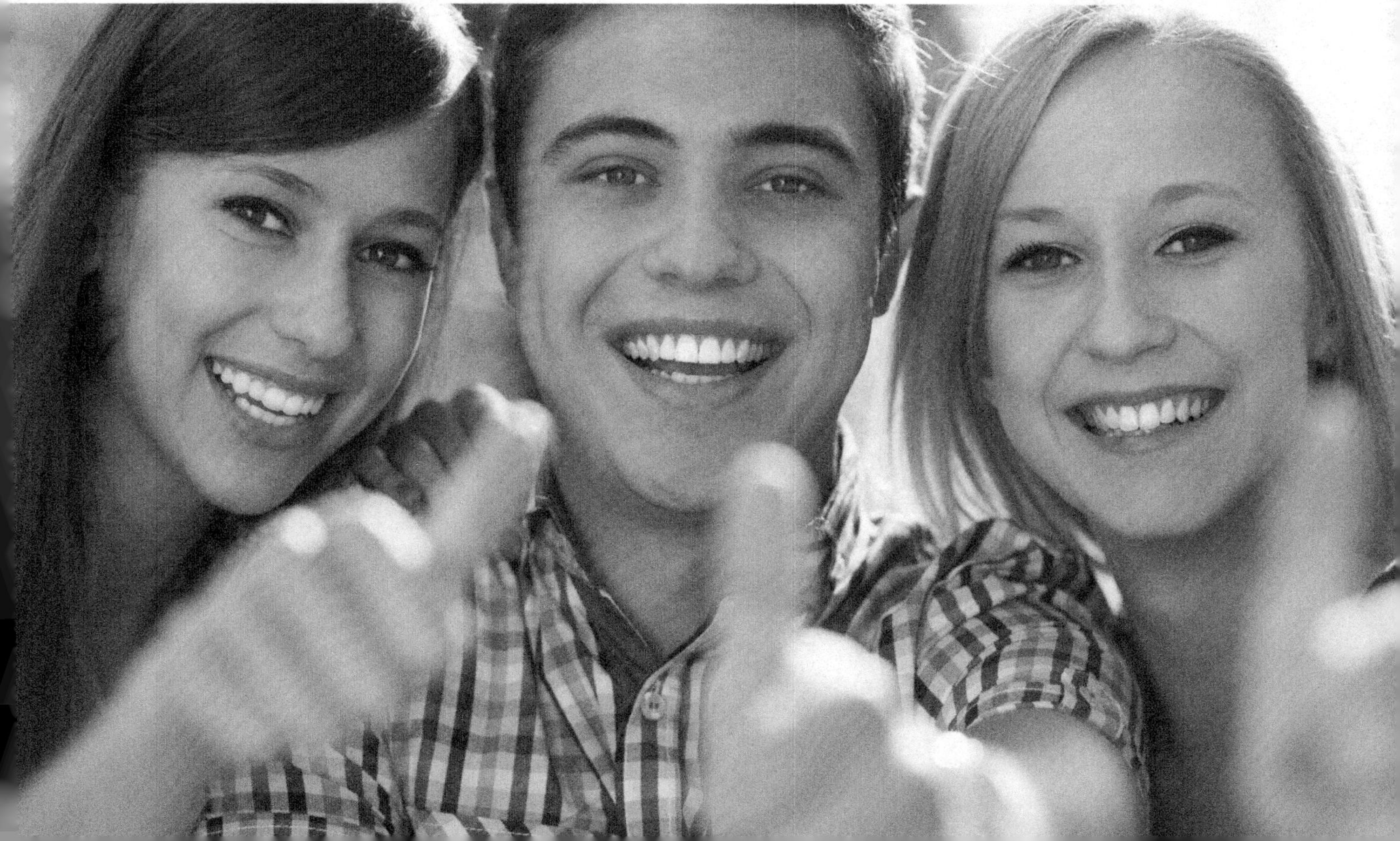

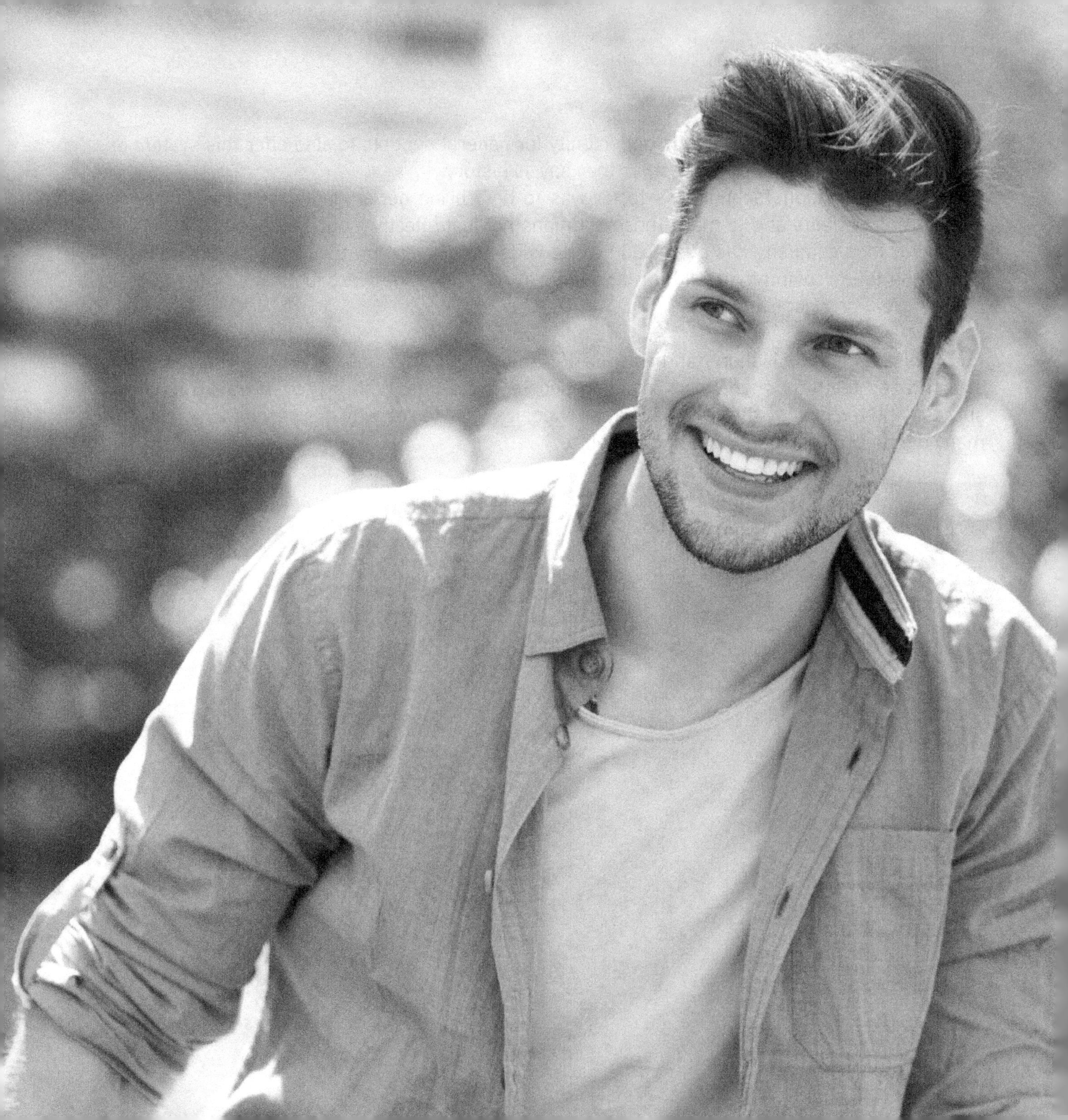

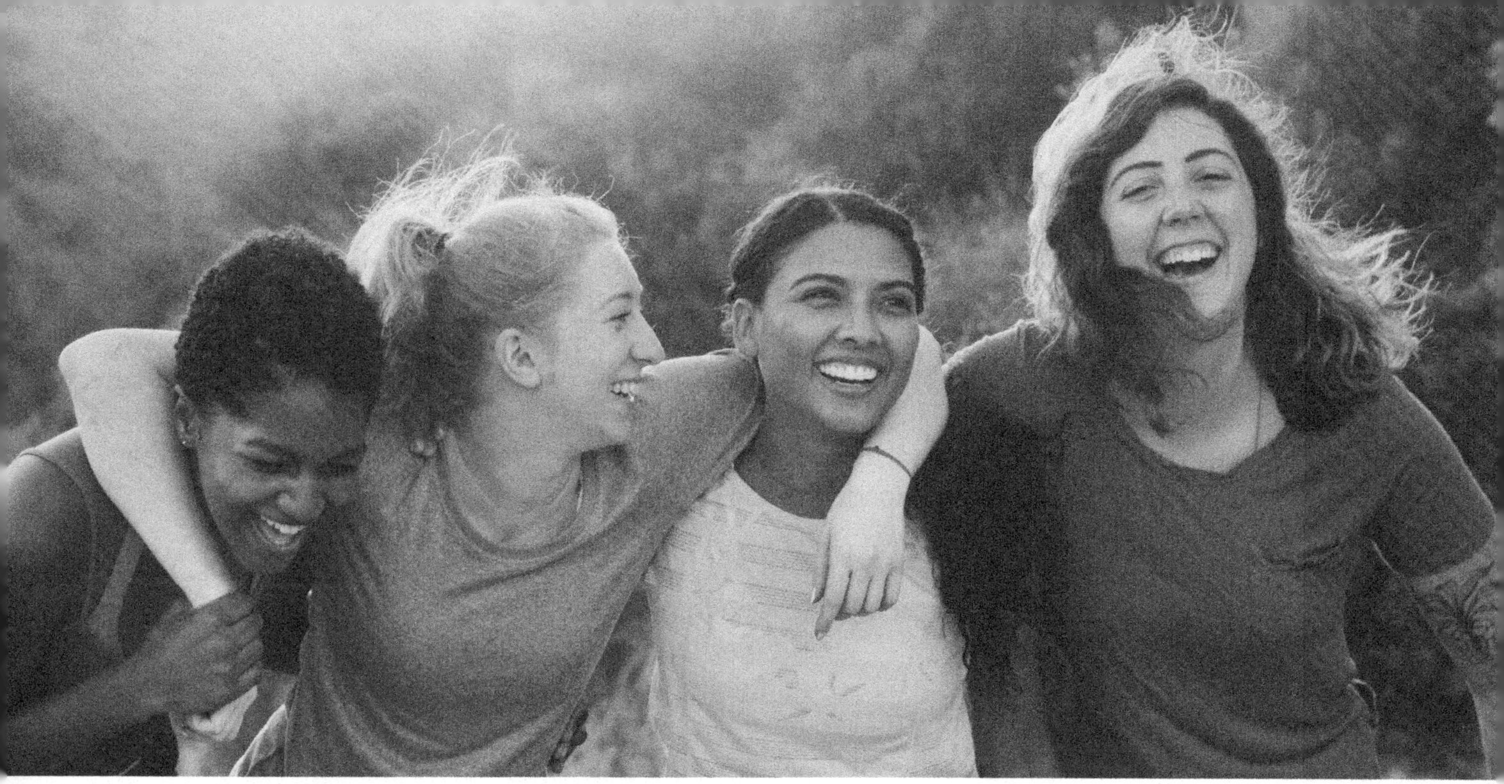

Invisalign Overview

Invisalign works using a system of clear aligner trays that are custom created to specifically fit your teeth. These trays are designed to be placed on both the upper and lower portions of your teeth. They are similar to a retainer (which is designed to keep teeth from shifting out of place). Each tray is designed to properly align your teeth into a beautiful and straight smile.

Aligner trays are switched out for new ones throughout the teeth straightening process, approximately every two weeks. Each tray works to reposition your teeth incrementally, so the process of switching out your trays for new ones will continue until the desired effects are achieved.

How long treatment lasts varies on the patient and the complexity of the problem being corrected. The average patient can expect to be in treatment for anywhere from six months on the less severe scale to 18 months for more serious cases.

It is recommended that a patient wear Invisalign aligners for approximately 22 hours a day. Your aligners are designed be working full time to move your teeth gradually, therefore, you must keep them in as much as possible - even when you are sleeping - so they can work effectively.

One of the dangers of not wearing your aligners as directed is that if you are not wearing them enough every day, your teeth will not be ready for the next tray in your treatment series because they will not be in the correct position. This will require you to be evaluated further to make sure that the process is working, and it also means that your treatment will have to be altered so that you are wearing the aligners for a longer period of time.

Part of the benefit of Invisalign is of course that unlike metal braces, they ARE removable. Here are some situation where it is acceptable for you to remove your aligners for a short time:

Eating and Drinking

Because the aligner tray creates a barrier between your teeth and your food that you are eating, you cannot eat with Invisalign on. It is difficult or even impossible to chew while wearing aligners, and doing so runs the risk of damaging the appliance, rendering it ineffective. This rule applies

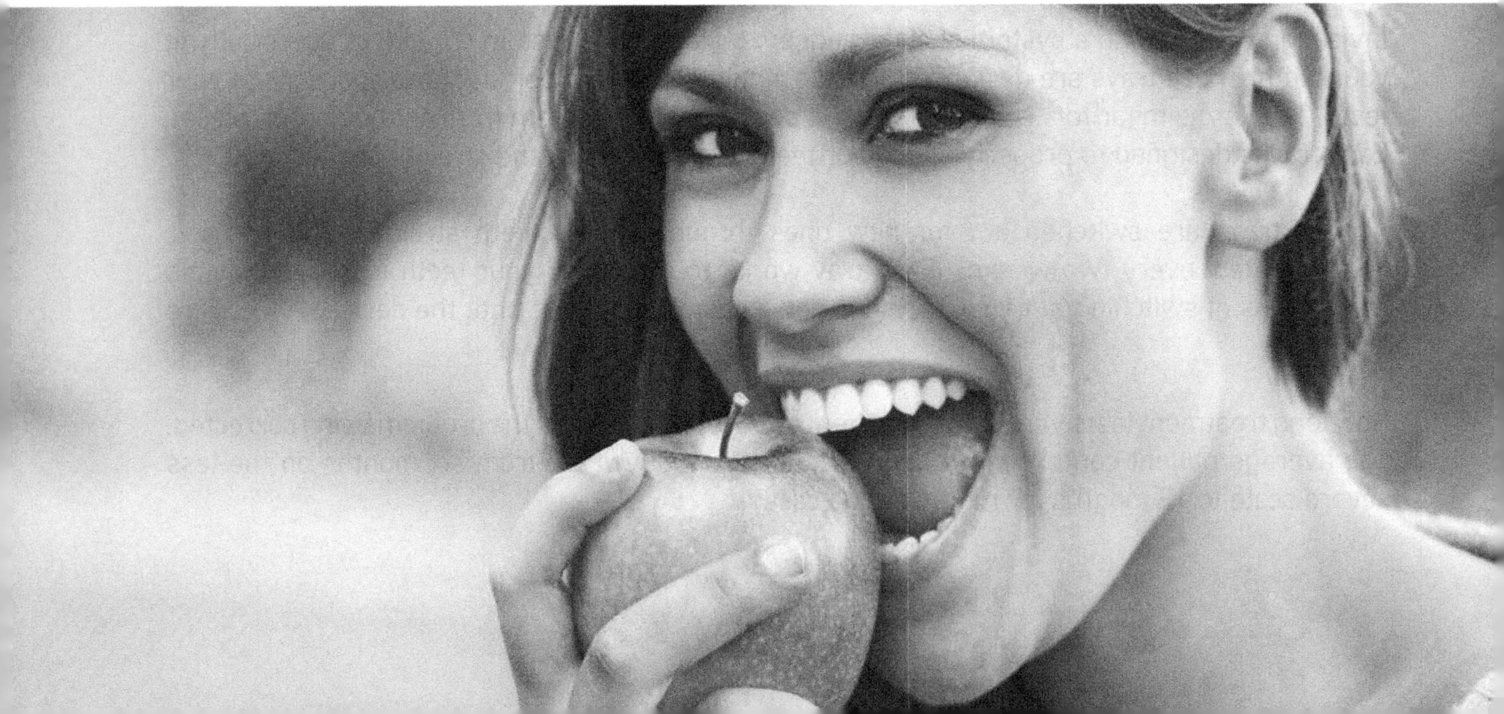

to things like candy, gum and lozenges as well. You should also remove your aligners before drinking anything besides water, as things like coffee can result in discoloration of your trays, and having sugary drinks or other similar substances trapped against your teeth by the aligners can damage your enamel.

Brushing and Flossing

Being able to keep up with your regular brushing and flossing/oral care routines without the added difficulty of brackets, braces and wires are a huge advantage that Invisalign has over traditional braces. When you are ready to brush and floss each day, remove your aligners and simply return them to your mouth as soon as you are done.

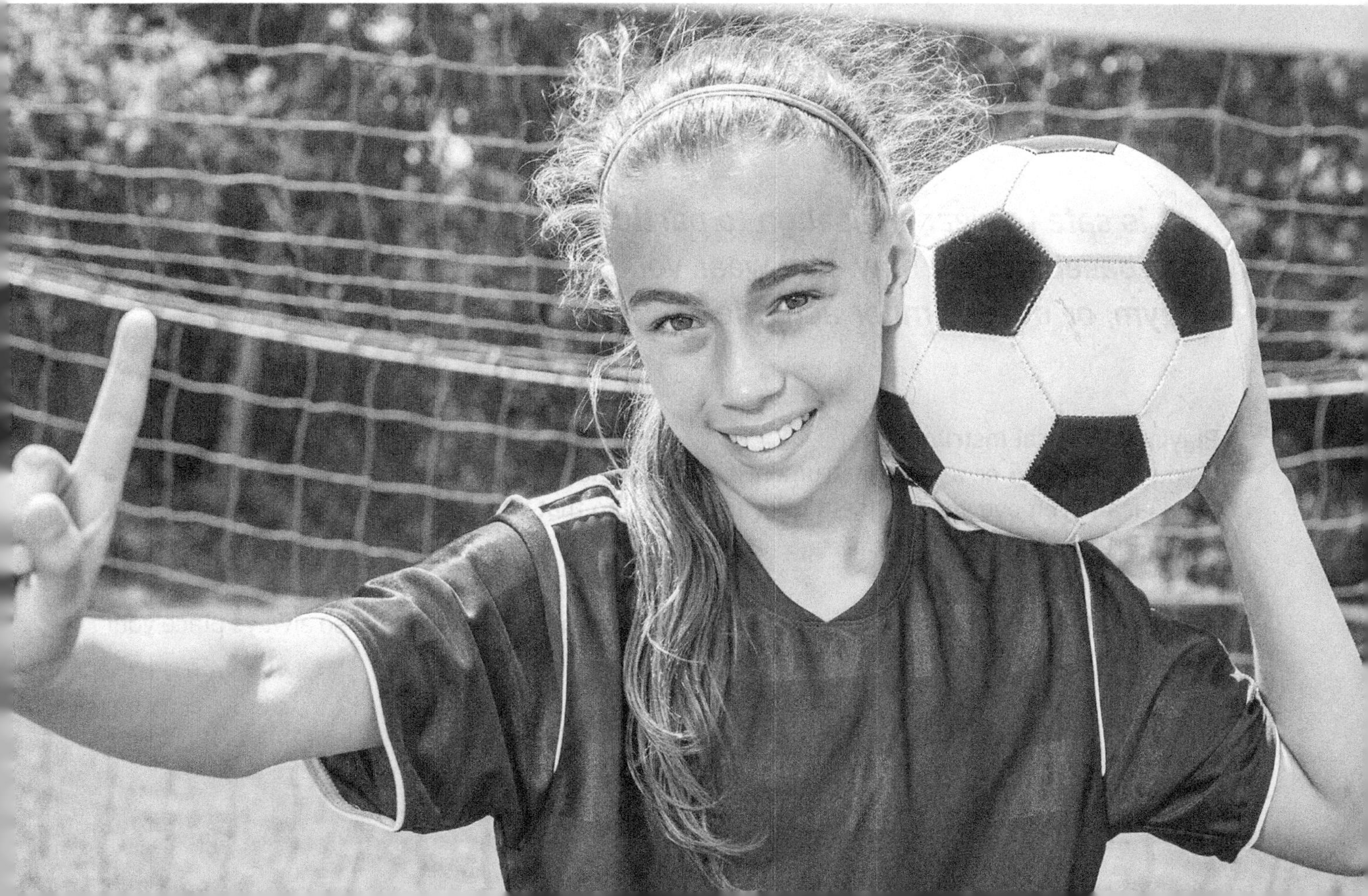

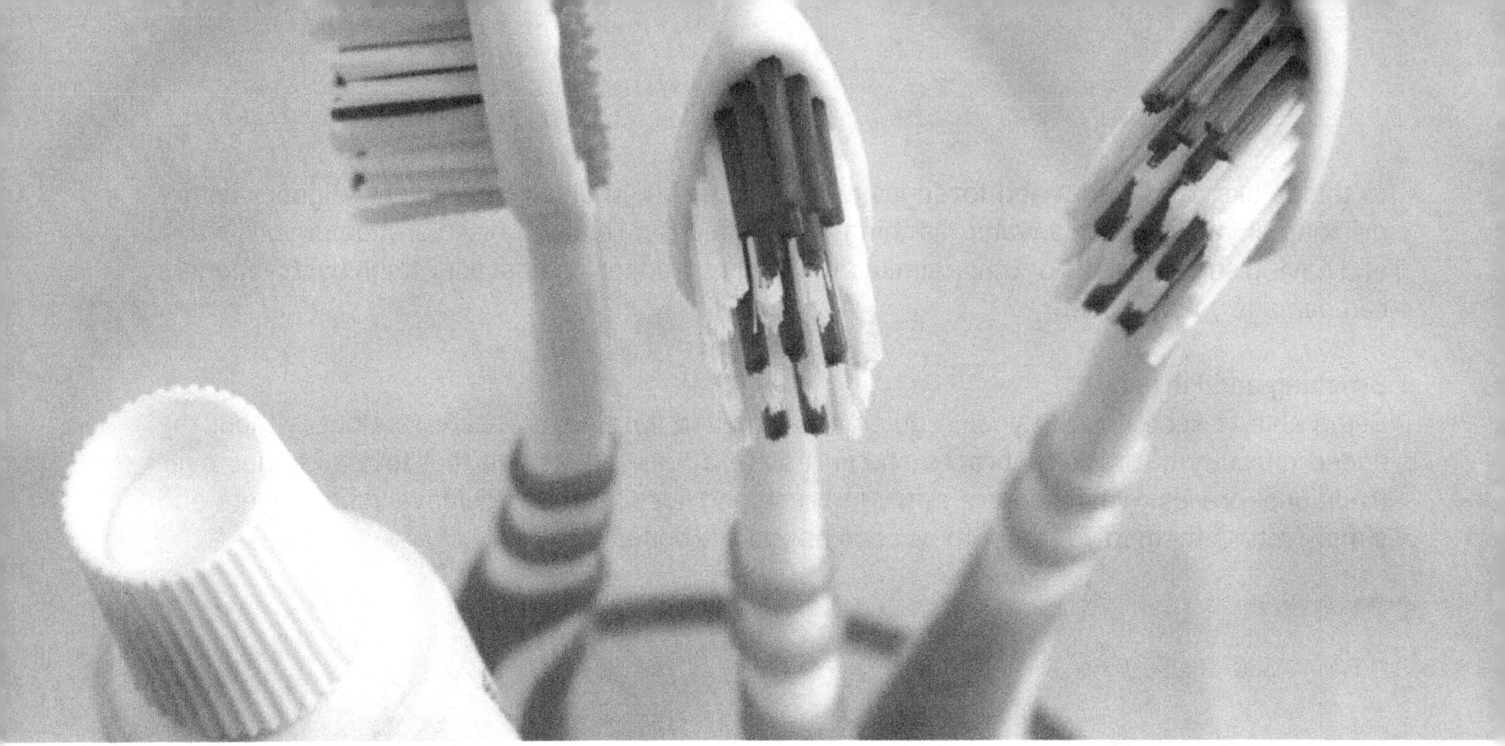

It is safe to wear Invisalign to participate in basketball, wrestling, or baseball. You may also wear your aligners when going to the gym, or other similar activities.

Playing a Musical Instrument

If you play a reed or a wind instrument such as a clarinet, the flute or the saxophone, it is a good idea to remove your aligners prior to playing so that you do not experience discomfort or damage your trays.

It is most efficient for your treatment to not damage or misplace your trays so always place your aligners in a safe place when they are not in your mouth.

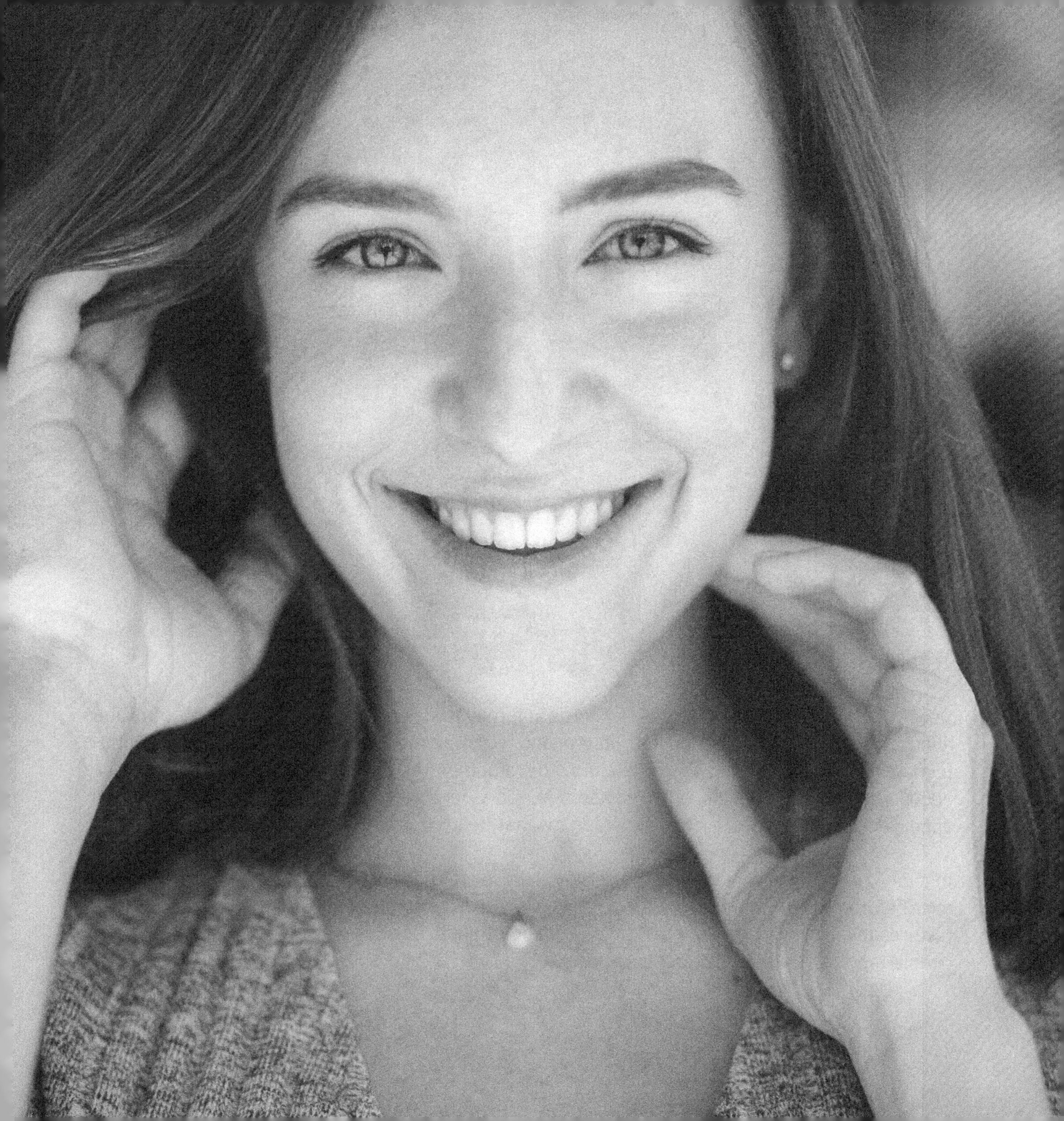

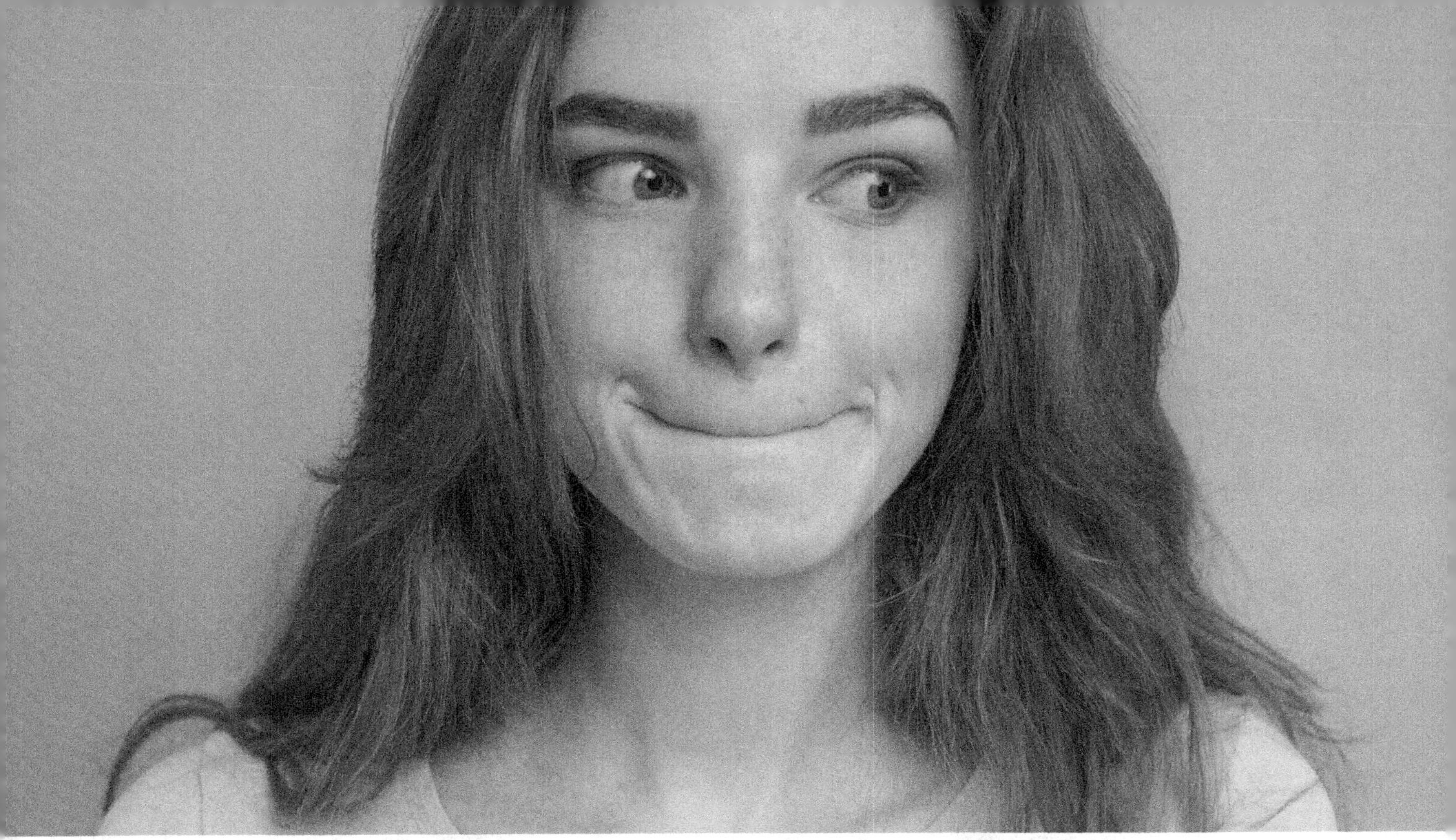

Treatment for Teens

Does your teen avoid taking selfies or photos at family functions because they are self conscious about their teeth? It is a common problem, and it can be more serious than you think. Being a teenager is very important time in a child's development as it is generally where their "future adult" personality is developed. It is also a period where they become far more aware of their appearance – and they are more sensitive to what their peers think of them.

In today's world, social media is prevalent and there are more photographs are being taken than ever before. No teen wants to be the boy or girl with crooked teeth in a group photo or in candid pictures taken as a school event which has the potential to be shared with friends, family or even people they don't know with just a few clicks.

Something like a few crooked teeth or an slight overbite might not seem like it is a big deal to an adult who has matured into knowing that, in the grand scheme of things, other people's opinions of us don't really matter much. But for a teen, these issues can be major factors that influence their self esteem. It can also be something that hinders their social skills and how they present themselves in things such as college interviews. In the long term, it can follow them to adulthood where they have to deal with job interviews, meetings and other situations where confidence is key to successful actions.

It goes without saying that all of this, combined with school, extracurricular activities, friends and even after school jobs, can make teenage years a very stressful time a young person's life. And while the path to resolving this may seem like simply getting your child braces to correct the problem, there are far more factors to consider than that.

Metal braces can correct a large percentage of issues with crooked teeth, spacing issues and other dental irregularities. But they also have a factor that can make a teen hesitant about pursuing orthodontic treatment that may they truly need - they are highly visible. While there is less stigma in recent years than in the past about wearing braces, adding ones that everyone can see to the mix when you have a teen who is already self-conscious can end up doing more harm than good.

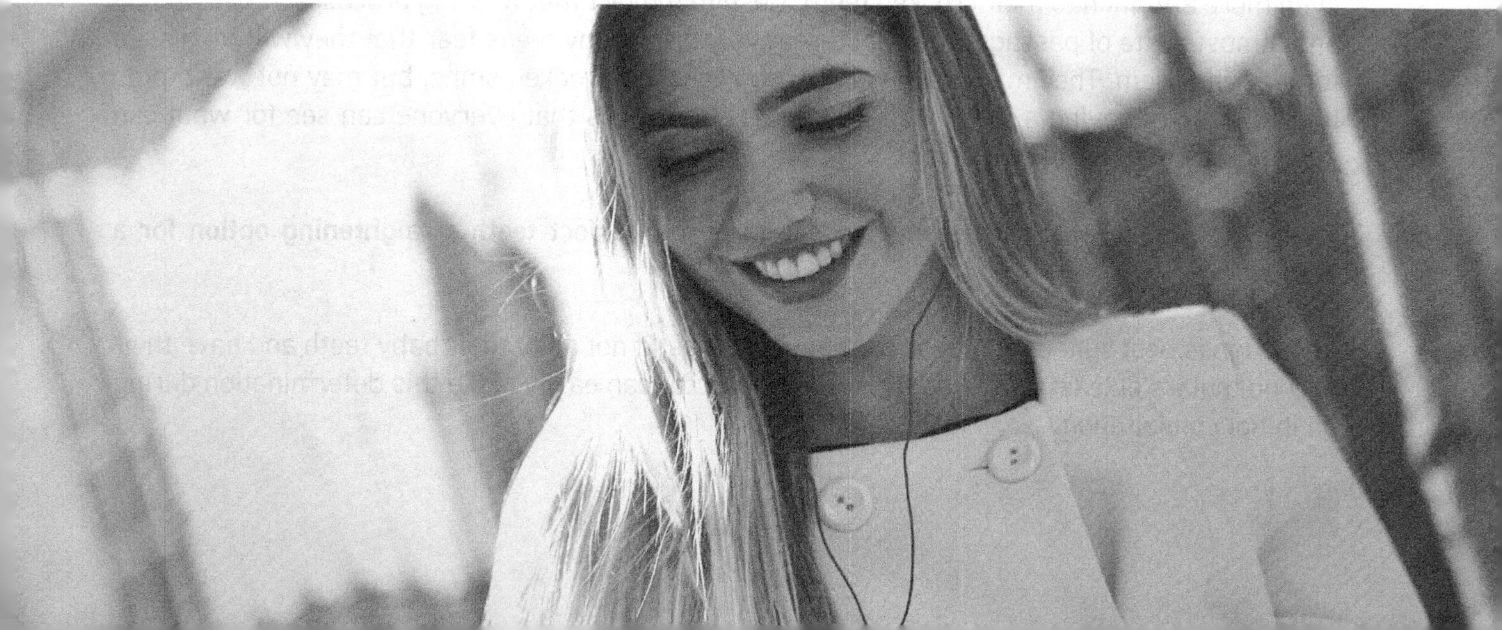

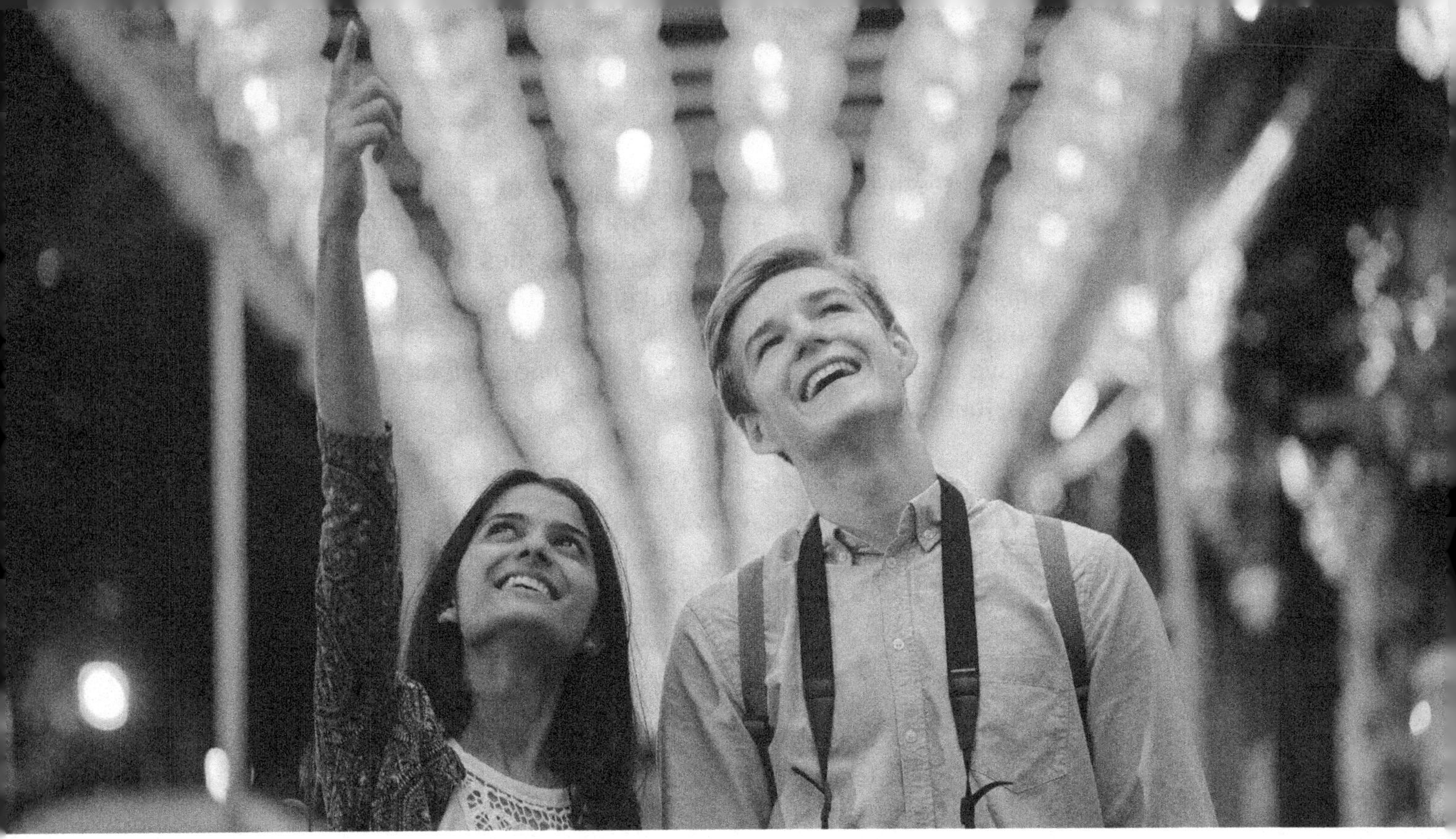

Putting metal braces on a teen's teeth can be demoralizing as many feel that it is attracting even more attention to their crooked teeth. Despite the fact that wearing braces is very common and almost a rite of passage for your formative years, many teens fear that they will be teased for wearing them. They may really want to correct their crooked smile, but may not want to do it at the risk of having a mouth full of brackets and wires that everyone can see for what can sometimes amount to several years.

These are just a few reasons why Invisalign is the perfect teeth straightening option for a teenager.

Invisalign is best suited for teens who have lost most if not all of their baby teeth and have their second molars at least partially erupted. Your doctor can easily make this determination during an initial consultation.

Invisalign Teen clear aligners work similarly to the way that the adult version does - the trays are created specifically for your teen's teeth using the same 3D technology which we will discuss later in this book. Each aligner is worn for approximately two weeks and each will work to straighten your teeth's teeth gradually until they achieve a straight, beautiful smile - without anyone noticing!

In addition to being clear and not easily detected, Invisalign also offers minimal amount of disruption to a teen's life. Most of today's teens lead a busy life filled with activities, sports, friends and family obligations. Orthodontic treatment with Invisalign requires less dental appointments, which most teens will welcome since it's certain that no teen's idea of fun is spending an afternoon sitting around at the orthodontist's office.

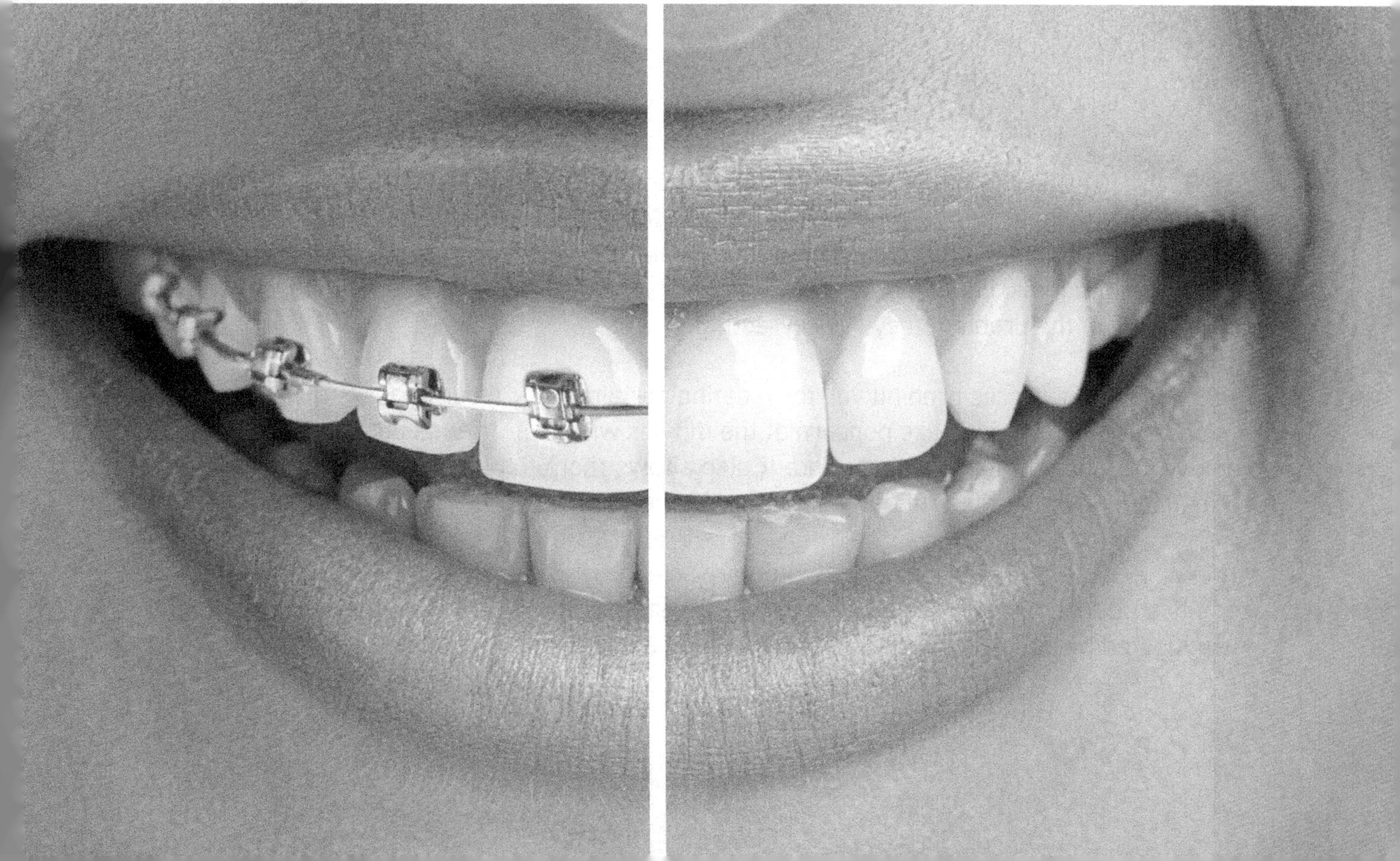

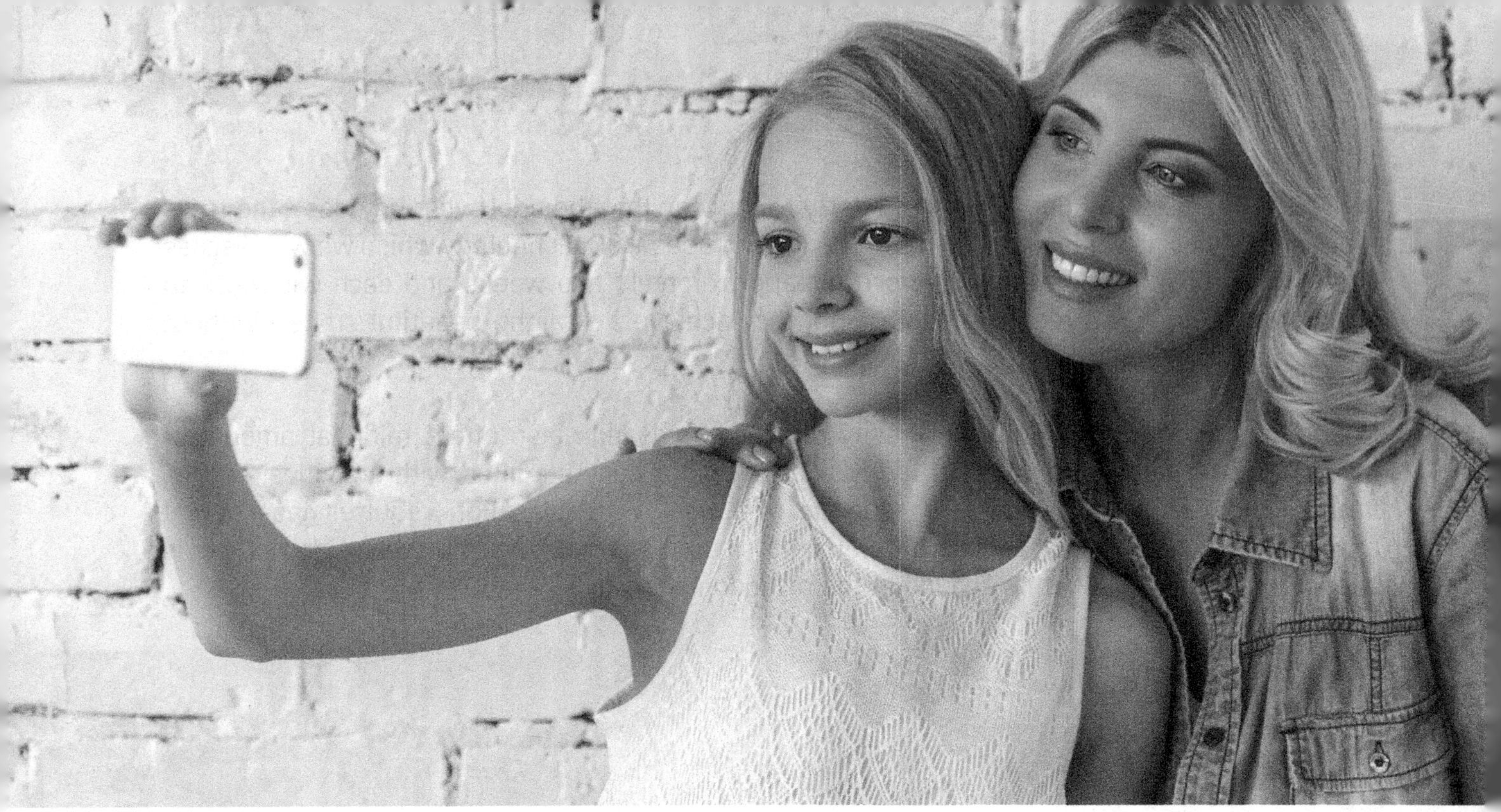

Treatment with Invisalign also offers a faster path for a teen to achieve the smile of their dreams. While traditional metal braces can sometimes require several years of permanent, daily wear – treatment with Invisalign generally takes about a year to 18 months to complete, depending on the severity of the problem they are correcting.

While traditional braces prohibit you from eating certain foods, clear aligners give your teen the option to still enjoy things like popcorn at the movies with their friends because they can simple remove the aligners for a short period. It also allows them to play their favorite sports of play an instrument without fear of damaging their braces.

Another benefit to Invisalign is that the care, cleaning and upkeep of aligners is much less complicated than metal braces. This will make it easy for a teen to follow the care regiment that is suggested by the orthodontist, and will not add a large time investment to their day.

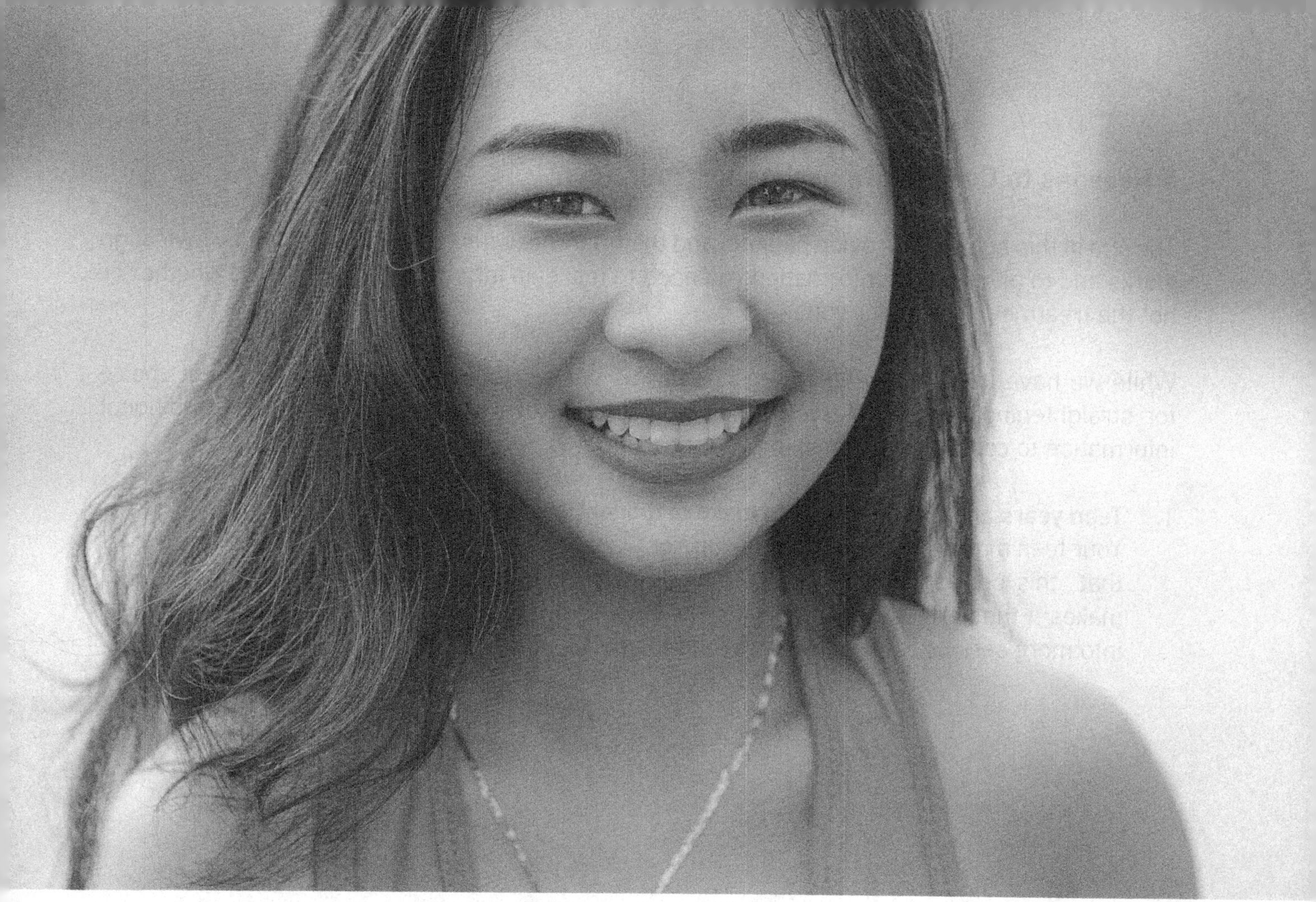

Having a healthy, beautiful smile is also not just about aesthetics. Having teeth which are straight are also easier to take care of, and makes you less susceptible to dental problems later in life, such as gum disease, problems with chewing, and even chronic headaches and pain issues.

Having a healthy level of self esteem as a teen is a key factor in how that teen's future is shaped. Every parent wants the best for their child - and wants them to grow into a healthy, productive and well adjusted adult. Helping your teen obtain a straight, healthy smile that they are proud of is an excellent way to start!

5 Reasons to Consider Invisalign for Your Teen

The aim of this book is to provide patients and their parents with knowledge about how Invisalign works and to give you the information you need to make an informed decision about whether or not the treatment is right for you.

While we have listed many other reasons in this section for why Invisalign is a great choice for straightening your teen's teeth, the five points below provide you with some additional information to consider when making your decision.

1. **Teen years are a perfect time to make orthodontic corrections**
   Your teen may be in a hurry to grow up - or want to be seen as "adult-like" - but the reality is that this period of their lives is one where they are still growing and developing. That makes it the perfect time to take care of issues with their teeth which, if ignored, can turn into more serious issues down the road to adulthood.

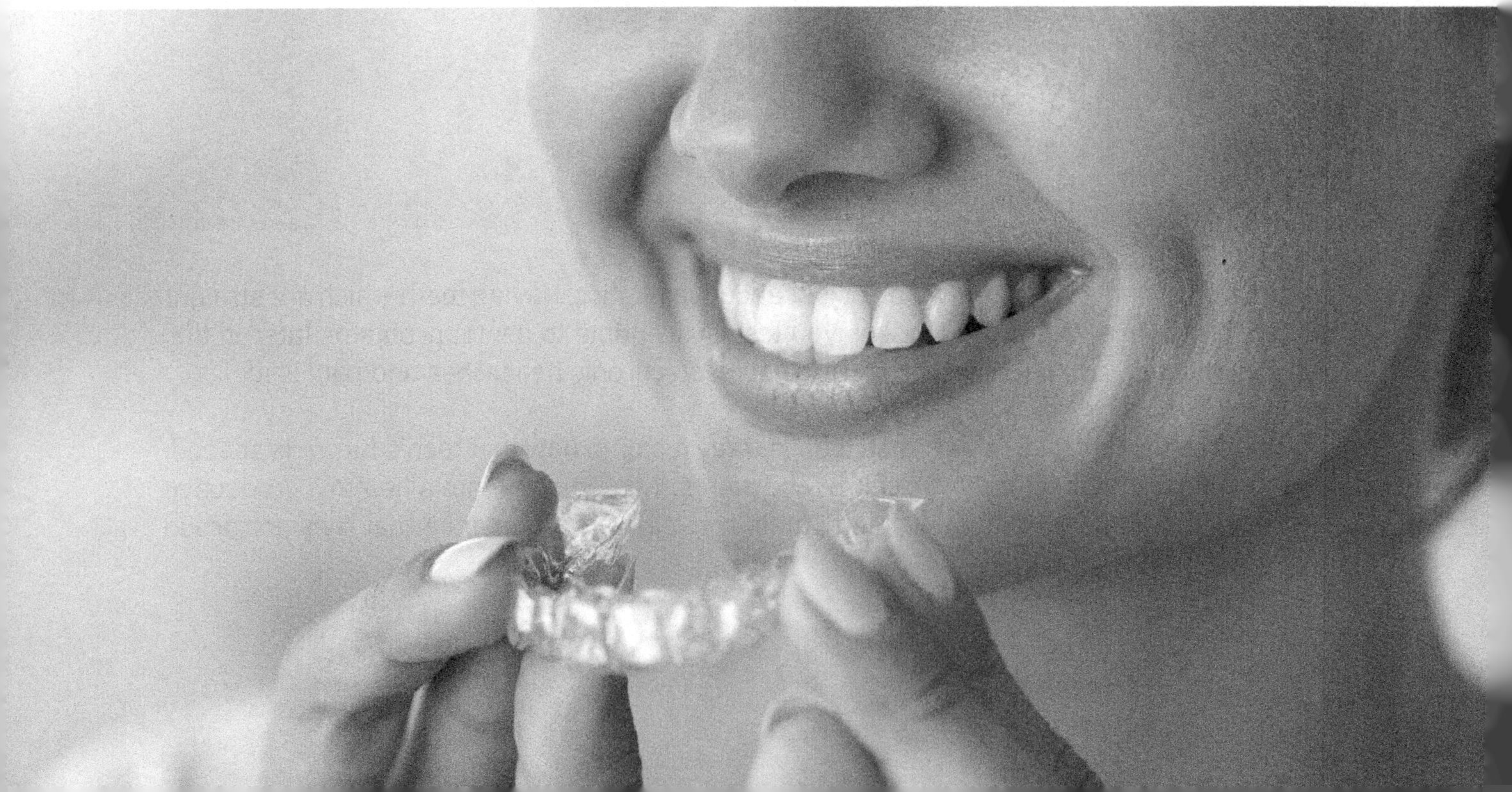

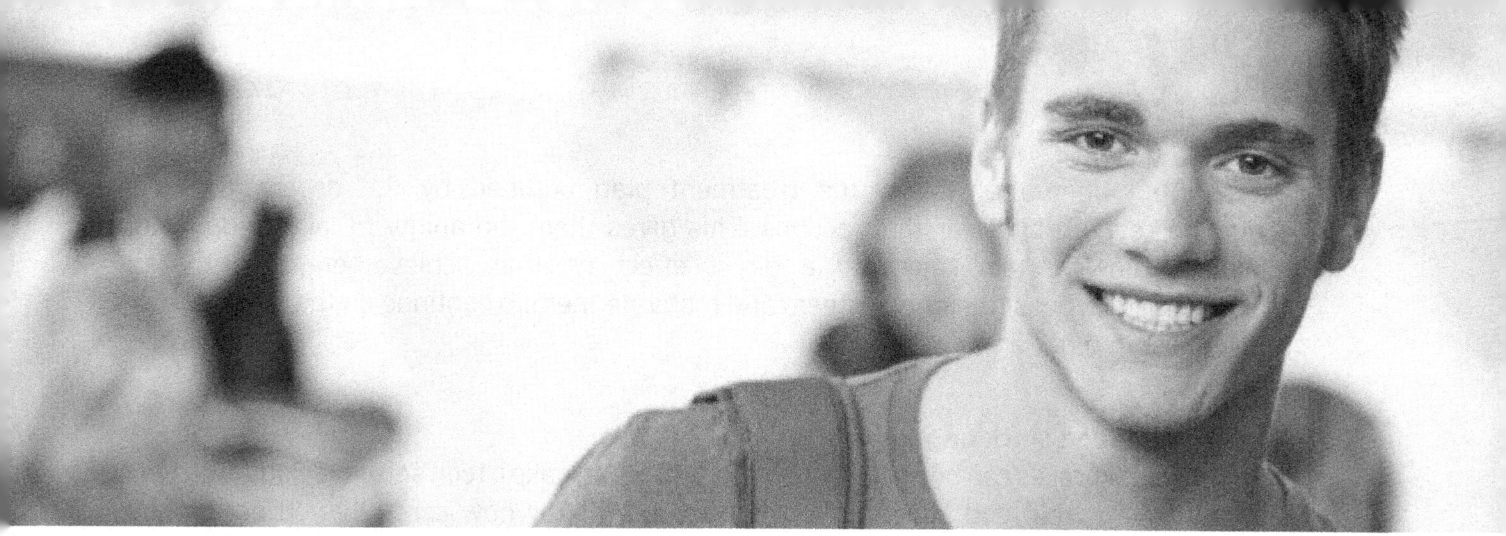

It is possible to use Invisalign for treatment as early as 11-12, but the average patient using is around 13-17. There are several factors which must be accounted for, such as baby teeth and the eruption of permanent incisors and first molars There cannot be the presence of significant tooth decay or damage. Your doctor can assist with determining if your child meets the criteria necessary to start treatment.

TS Orthodontics is one of NC's top Invisalign providers. Please contact us at 828-254-4602 or visit our website at www.mytsosmile.com to set up your complimentary Smile Assessment.

2. **It provides your teen with responsibility**
   Giving your teen a responsibility and showing them that they are in charge of things in their life is an excellent self-esteem booster. Taking charge of responsibilities is also a very valuable life skill.

   While you can certainly supervise them and provide them with reminders, it is ultimately up to the teen to comply with their recommended treatment and in turn, benefit from it's results. When they follow the treatment plan outlined by the doctor, they are assuming responsibility for their actions. This gives them the ability to take pride in the outcome, knowing that they had a direct effect on that achievement, and that is bound to further boost their self esteem and motivate them to continue on the path of being responsible in other areas too.

3. **No danger of food stuck on your braces**

   Wearing metal braces can be not just uncomfortable and make a teen self conscious, but it can also leave you with food stuck on your braces no matter how carefully you eat or how specifically you follow your doctor's instructions on what you can and cannot eat. Having food stuck on your braces can be embarrassing and add to the feeling of self-consciousness the teen may feel about wearing braces in the first place. Not to mention that it is far more difficult to brush your teeth with metal braces and that can lead to frustration.

   These things are never an issue with Invisalign. Teens never have to worry about cleaning off their braces because you can simply remove them to eat and to brush their teeth, making it easy to eat the things they like and keep up with their oral hygiene routines.

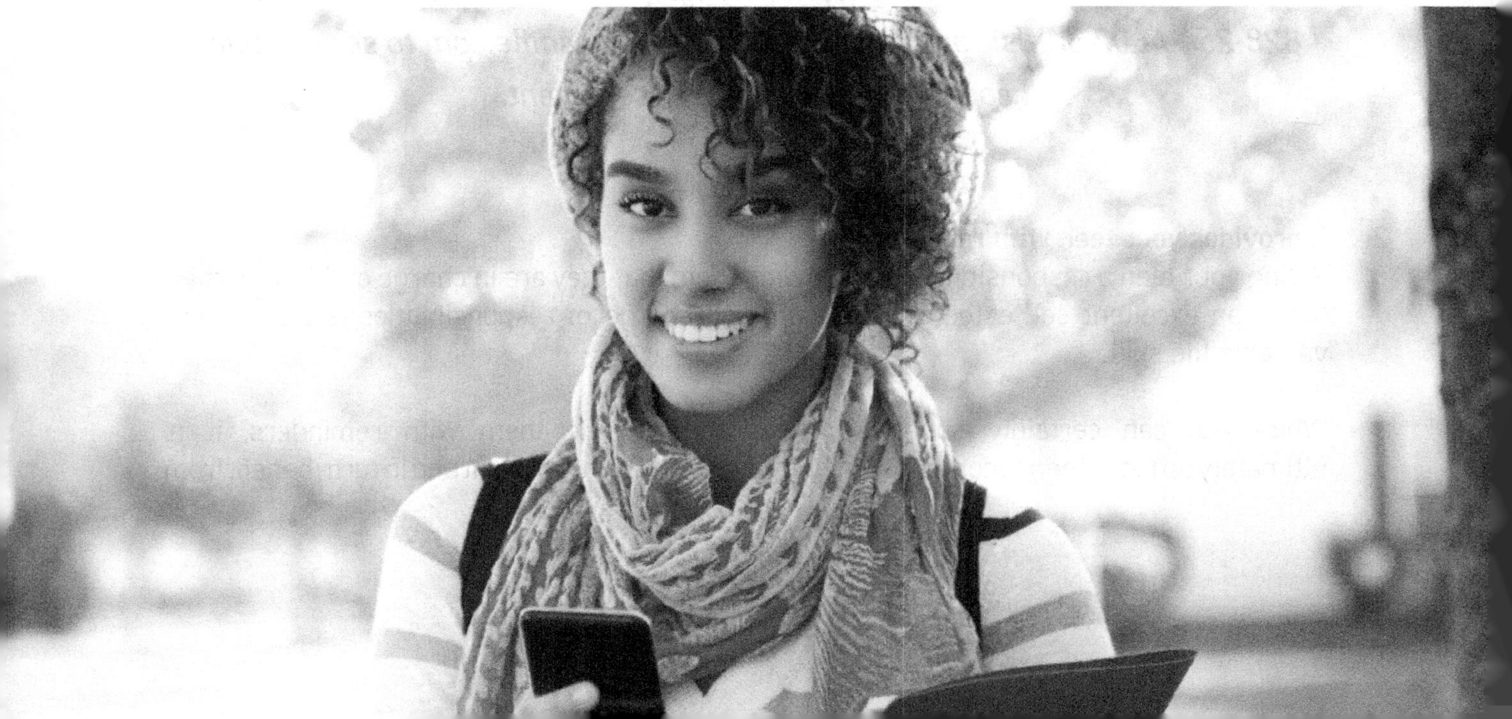

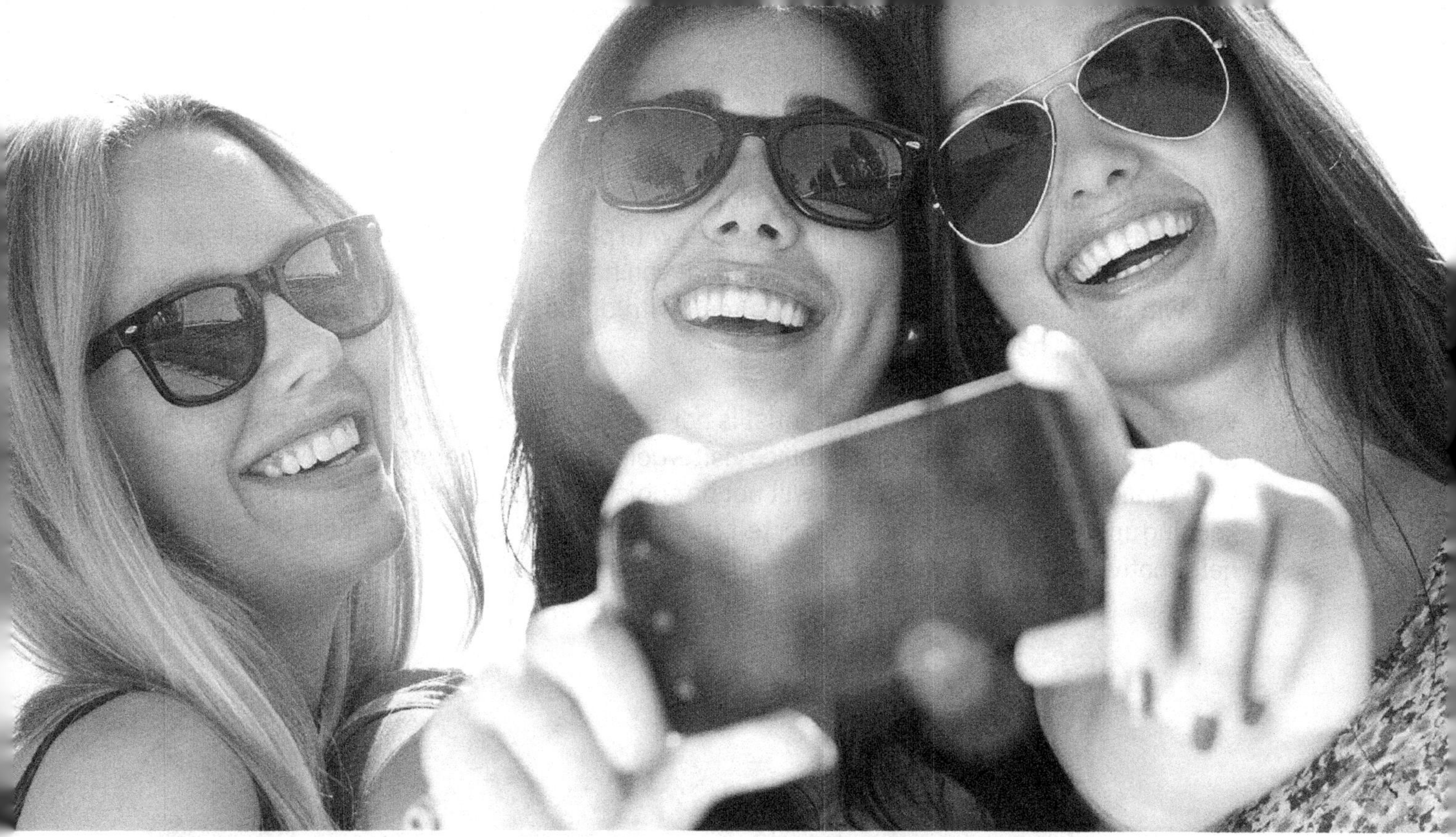

4. **More comfortable than any other alternatives to metal braces**
One of patient's greatest and most common anxieties about getting braces is pain and discomfort in both putting the braces on, living with them every day, and removing them. This is in addition to already being worried about their appearance, so needless to say even the idea of these things can be very stressful for a teen.

With Invisalign, your teen does not need to worry about looking or feeling their best since the aligners are virtually undetectable during daily use. The gum, jaw and tooth pain that people commonly associate with wearing braces is also eliminated, as Invisalign is extremely comfortable to wear and does not cause any discomfort once you are accustomed to wearing your aligners. It provides an over all better and more pleasant experience for getting the smile that you want...without having pain that you don't!

5. **No fear of going to the dentist or orthodontist**
   People generally associate going to the dentist with pain and discomfort, and this is especially the case when you wear braces. Knowing that you have an orthodontist's appointment - and you will have many to follow - can fill a teen with dread and they may do anything in their power to avoid having to go.

   With Invisalign, a trip to the orthodontist is not scary, and your teen will learn this very early on in the process. They know that an office visit is going to be routine so they can walk in the office with confidence, knowing that they will not be subjected to discomfort. And, if they have been keeping up with their treatment as directed, they will get some praise from the doctor, which will help motivate them to continue being diligent and responsible.

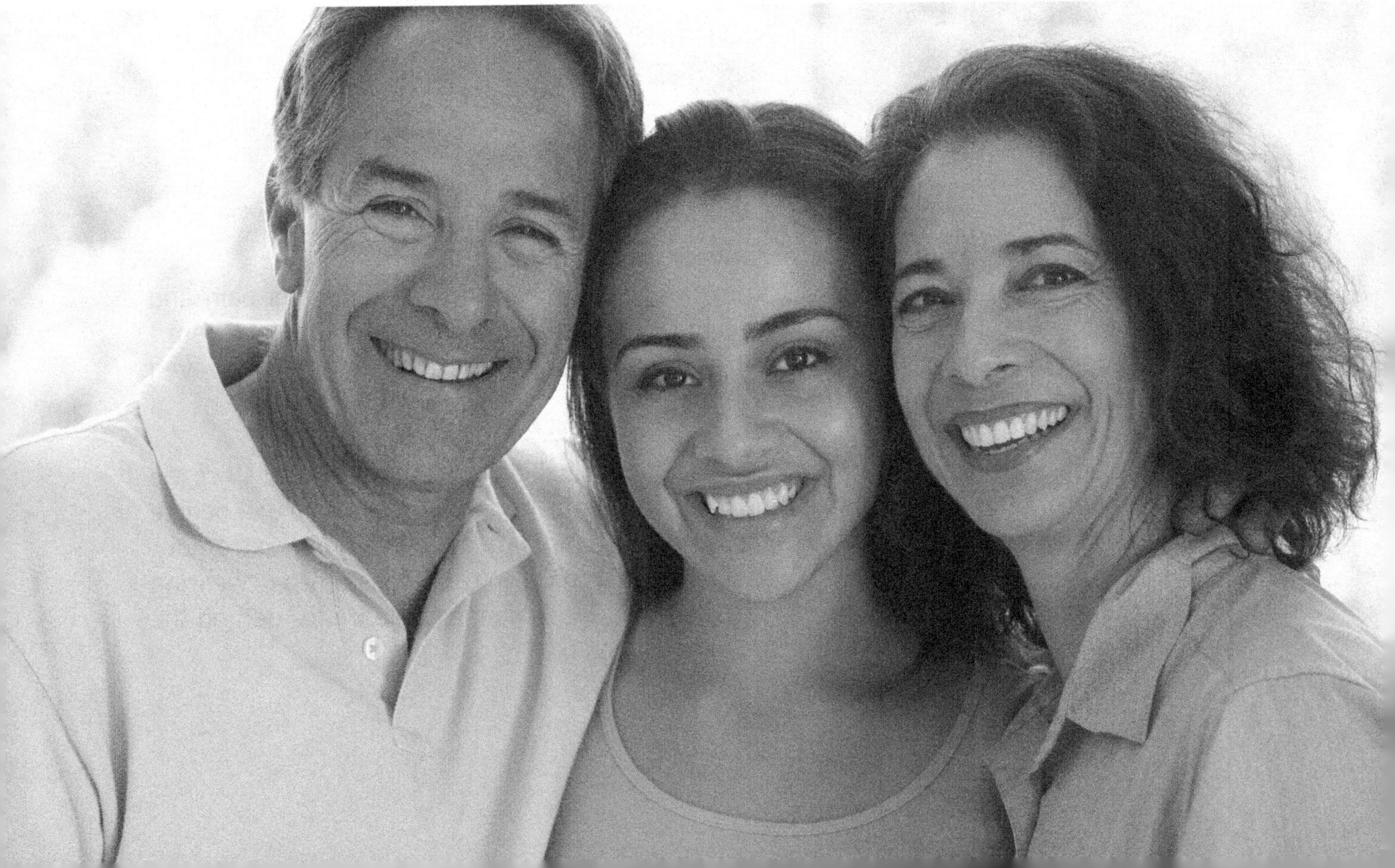

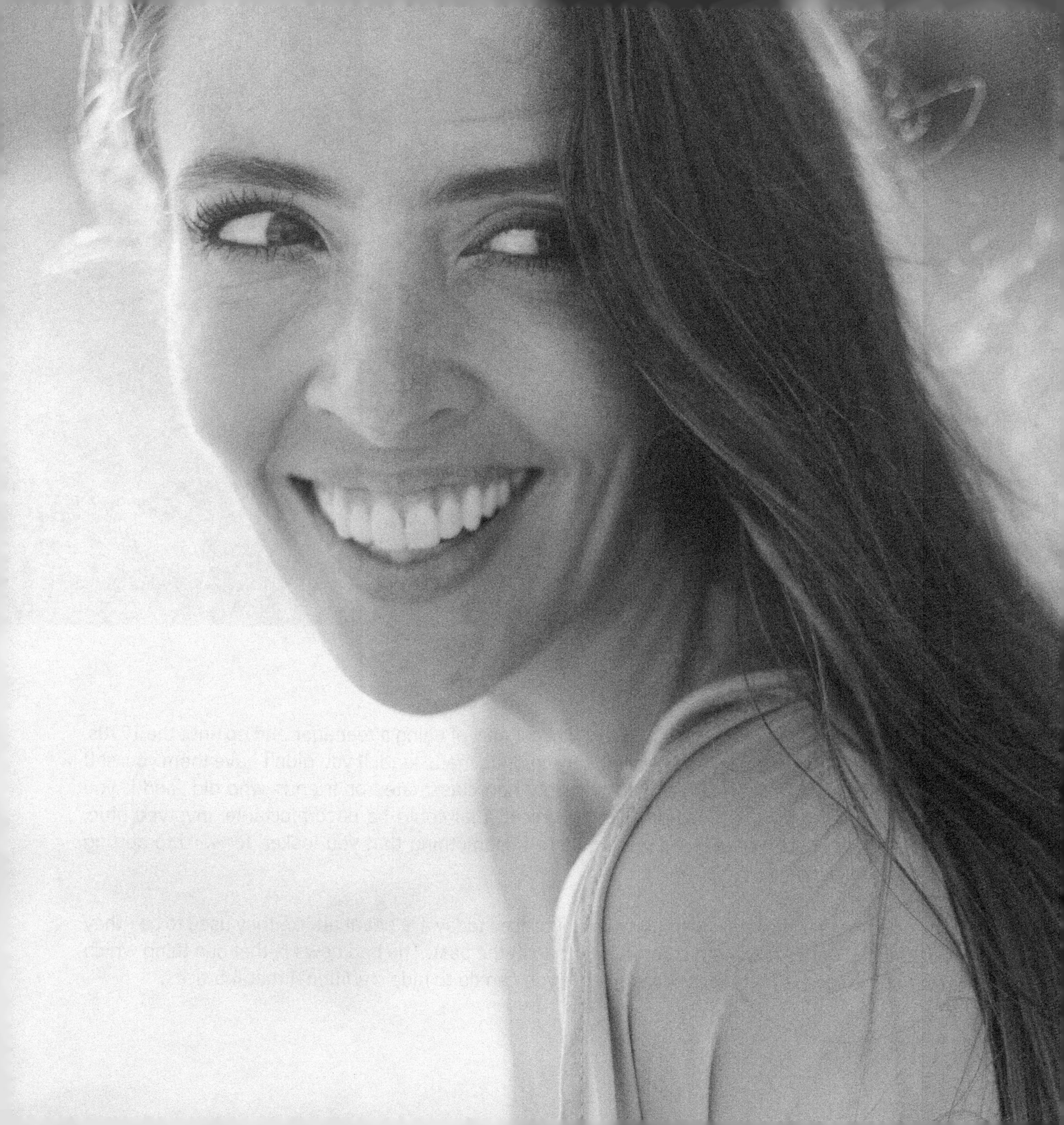

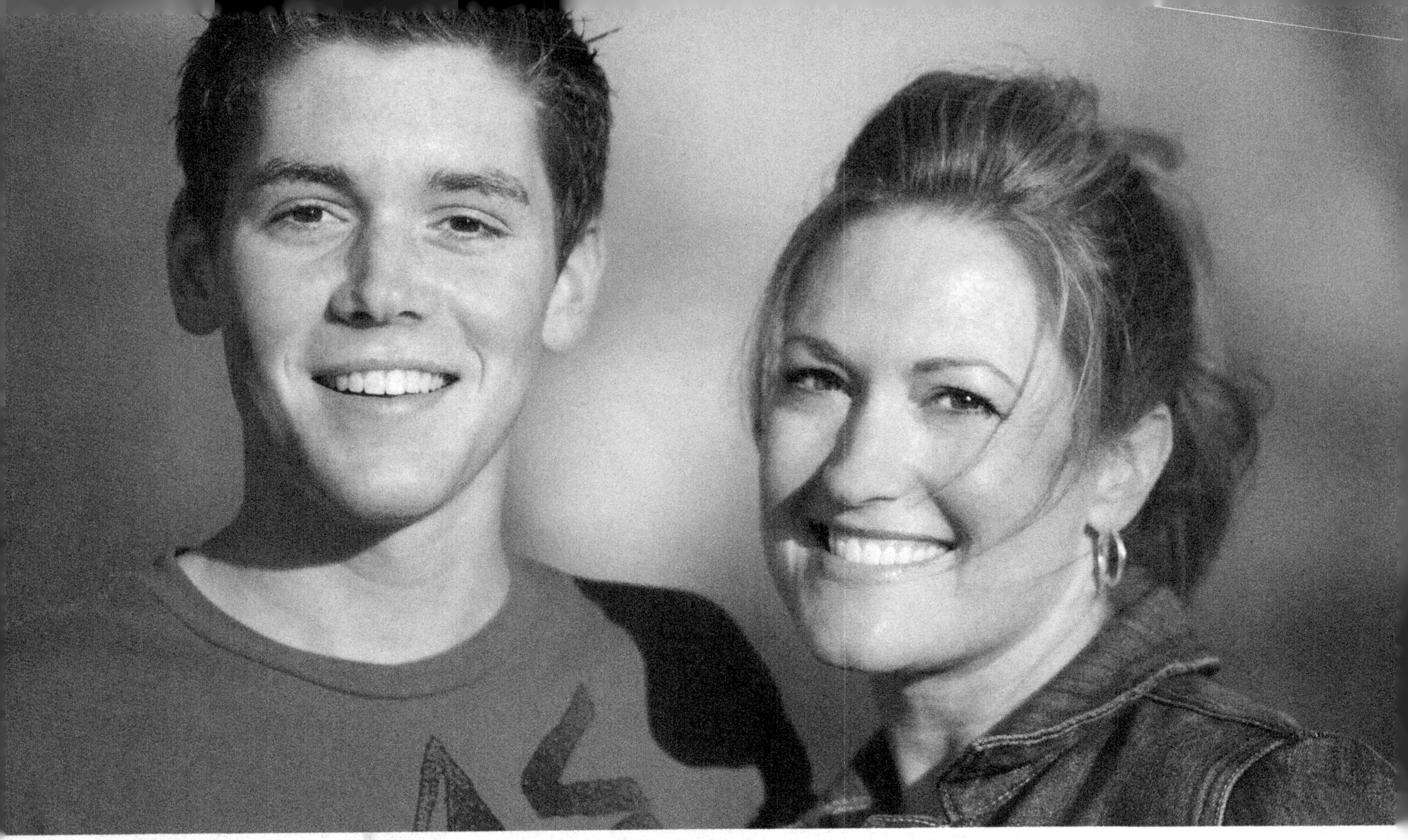

Information for Parents

For many years, braces have been a very normal part of being a teenager and up until the 1990s, the only type that was available were the traditional, metal kind. If you didn't have them yourself as a young person, chances are you probably had classmates or friends who did...and if you did personally wear them you are likely to recall that could be uncomfortable, involved glue, brackets and rubber bands, and were generally something that you looked forward to getting over and done with.

The good news is that even traditional metal braces today are not at all like they used to be - they are smaller, flatter and more comfortable than in the past. The bad news is that one thing which has not changed is that there is really little you can do to hide traditional metal braces.

As a parent, you always want to make sure you are making the choices which are best for your child and their well being. When you learn that your child needs braces, you will naturally have questions about treatment, what the best options are, how long it will take, and how much it will cost. In this book, we will discuss all of these things so that you can read it and know that you are making the right decision for your child's orthodontic treatment.

Even though braces have evolved over time and are very commonplace amongst young people, one thing that has not changed is that teens tend to feel self conscious wearing them. Being a teenager is difficult in today's world where a "sharing culture" exists and photographs are taken just about anywhere, anytime. Teens tend to be highly aware of the way they look when they reach that age, and naturally they want to look their best whenever these situations occur.

Having a physical imperfection such as a crooked smile can already make these kinds of moments socially uncomfortable - adding on metal braces that they feel only draws more attention to the problem can be demoralizing and have a serious impact on their already fragile self-esteem.

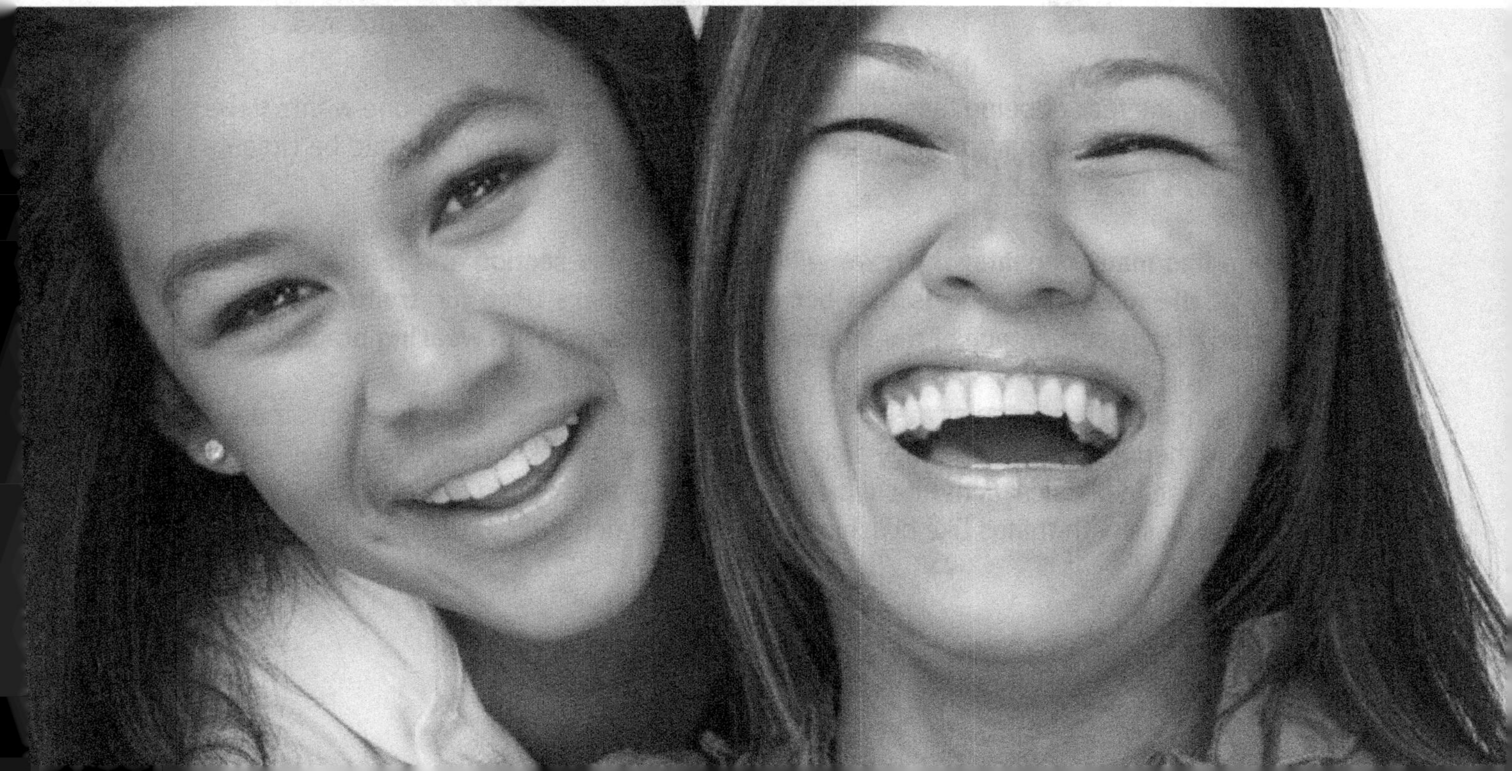

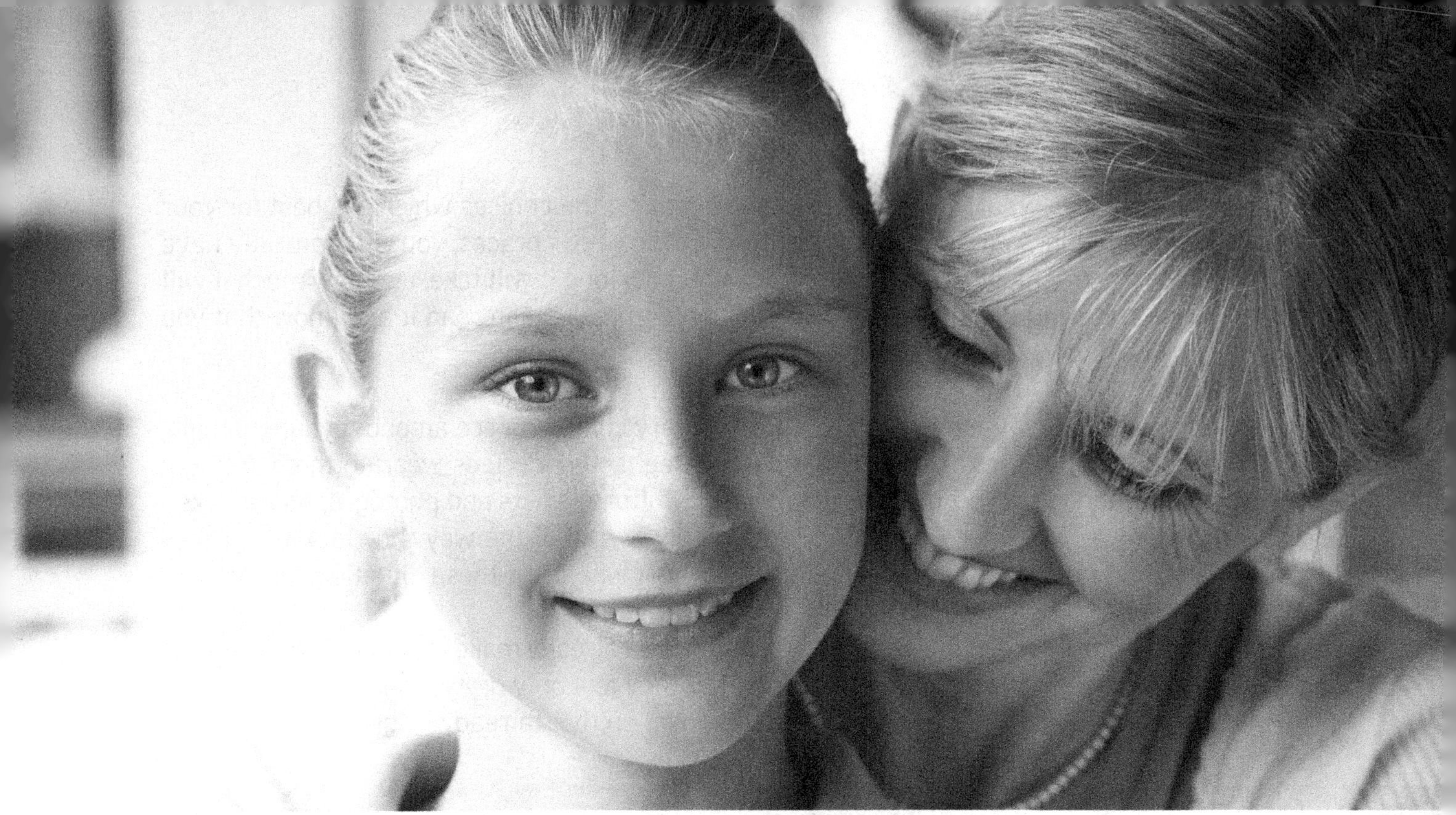

There is also the fear of being teased for wearing braces to consider. No one wants to be called "metal mouth" and as a parent, you naturally want to avoid having your child be ridiculed over their smile OR having braces.

Invisalign has many benefits which we will discuss in this section and throughout this book, but one of the most appealing is that because the aligners used for treatment are clear, it eliminates a large percentage of the stigma factor associated with wearing braces.

Between school, extracurricular activities, sports, friends and even part time jobs, today's teens have busy schedules. By nature, they also tend to take more risks. This means they will not only want to engage in physical activities which traditional braces would make difficult, but they will be more reckless with things like brushing, flossing and general dental hygiene.

Invisalign helps to address both of these issues as clean aligners are far safer when participating in sports or other physical activities.

It is also less painful and cumbersome to brush and floss with the obstacle of permanent braces. Having the option to remove the aligners for cleaning routines will encourage your teen to do it more often, and in turn instill good habits in them that they will take into adulthood.

Having aligners also allows the teen to still eat their favorite foods while they are in treatment. Things like eating popcorn when going to the movies with friends would be prohibited with traditional, metal braces. ***Not the case with Invisalign.*** Being able to participate in even a small activity like this has subtle positive benefits as they will not feel excluded from the things their friends are doing. That in turn helps them feel "normal" and not only better about themselves, but about their treatment process since it does not interrupt their daily life.

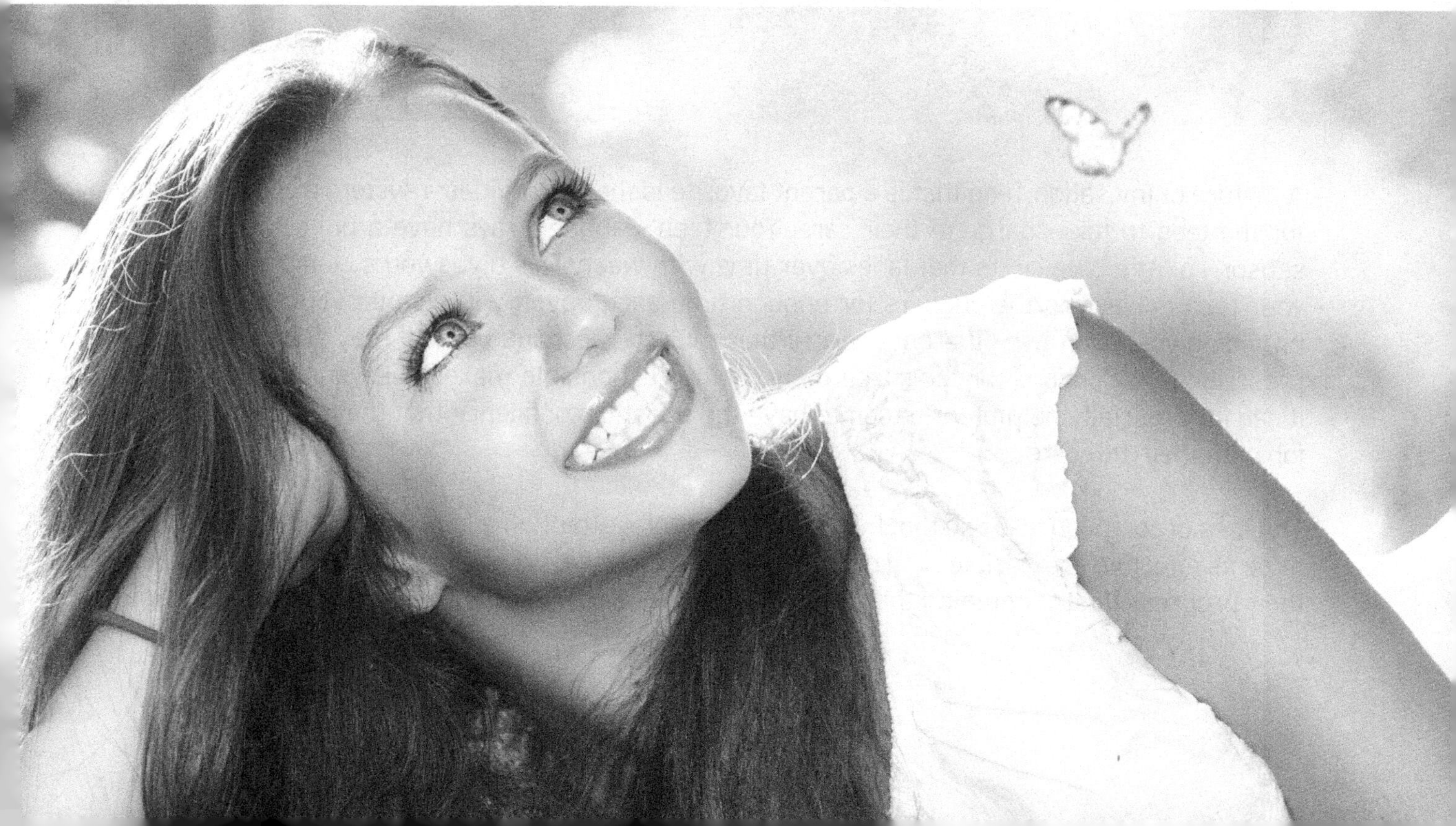

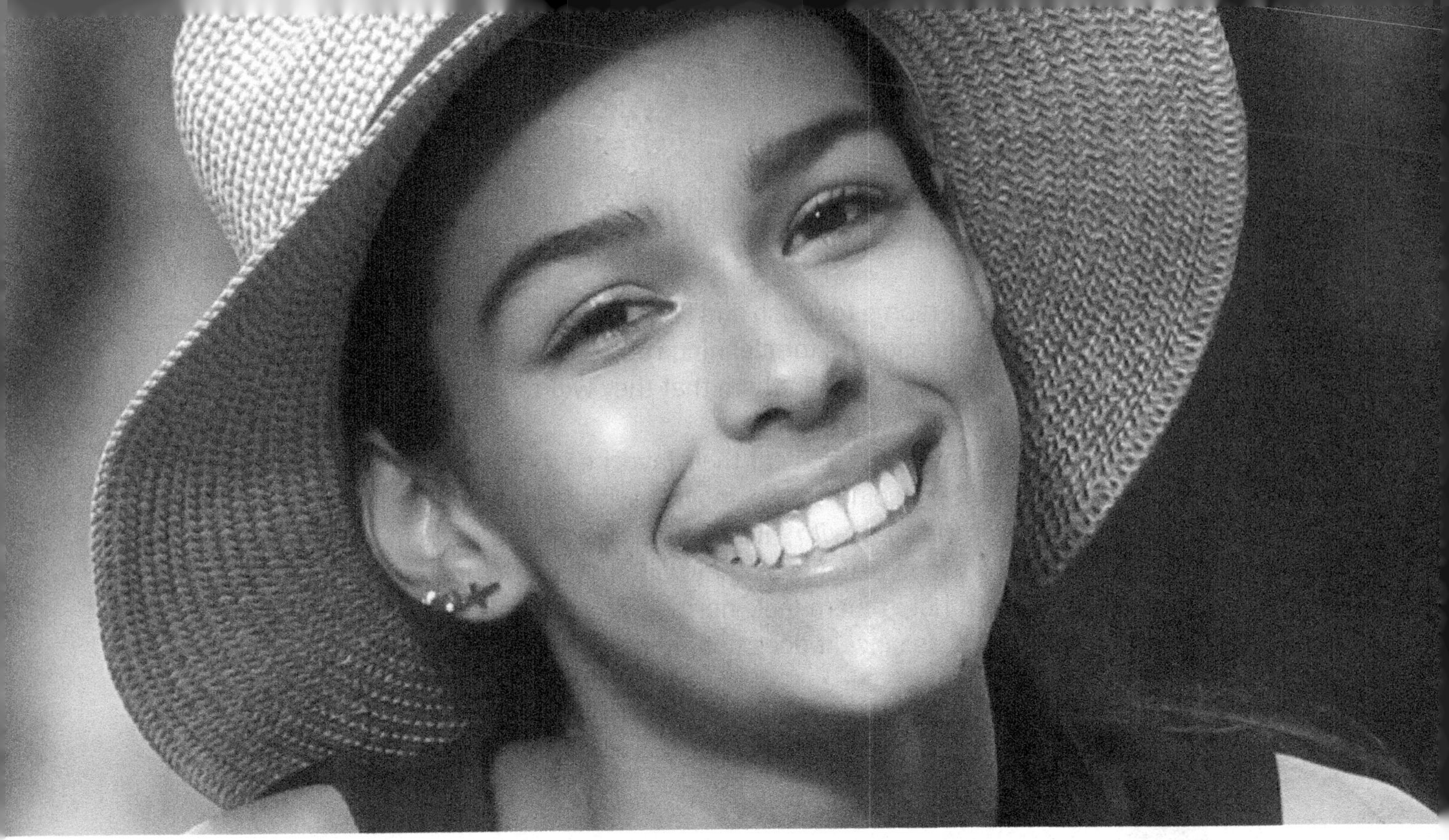

A feature of Invisalign Teen that is a parent favorite is that it provides a system of accountability for the teen to take charge of their care. Your teen's aligner trays have a built in compliance sensor - a little blue circle that fades over time with wear. This gives you a clear indicator that your teen is wearing the aligners for enough time each day. It will also let your doctor know, providing your teen two different sources they must be accountable to if they are not following prescribed instructions for their treatment. Being responsible makes everyone feel good, and it can be especially helpful for a teen to have the boost of confidence that they are doing a good job with their self care.

The area of compliance is one that may require parental attention and help in order for treatment to be as effective as possible. The biggest issue that we see amongst teen patients that hinders their progress in straightening their teeth is that they simply don't wear their aligners enough.

This is especially prevalent in the beginning of treatment, where there is a slight adjustment period for their first few trays. During this time, your teen may speak with a bit of a lisp, or notice that they are having an increase in saliva production as their mouth adjusts to having something new in it for an extended period of time. This can discourage them from wearing their aligners, even though they are made aware by the doctor that over time and regular wear, that this issue will go away. At this time, it's important as a parent to encourage your teen and support them - as well as help make sure they are wearing their aligners when that extra help is needed.

At this point, you may have decided that Invisalign is a good and viable option for your teen, but there is a caveat to consider: the maturity level of your child. This is actually a bigger issue than their actual age, because Invisalign requires a great deal of patient compliance and responsibility in order to be effective.

Most kids who undergo the treatment understand that it is a serious matter and have no problem with taking the responsibility, but all children are different. Children tend to be absent-minded by nature, and some are not as attentive as others. If your child struggles with these issues, they may need parental guidance to ensure that their treatment works as effectively as possible.

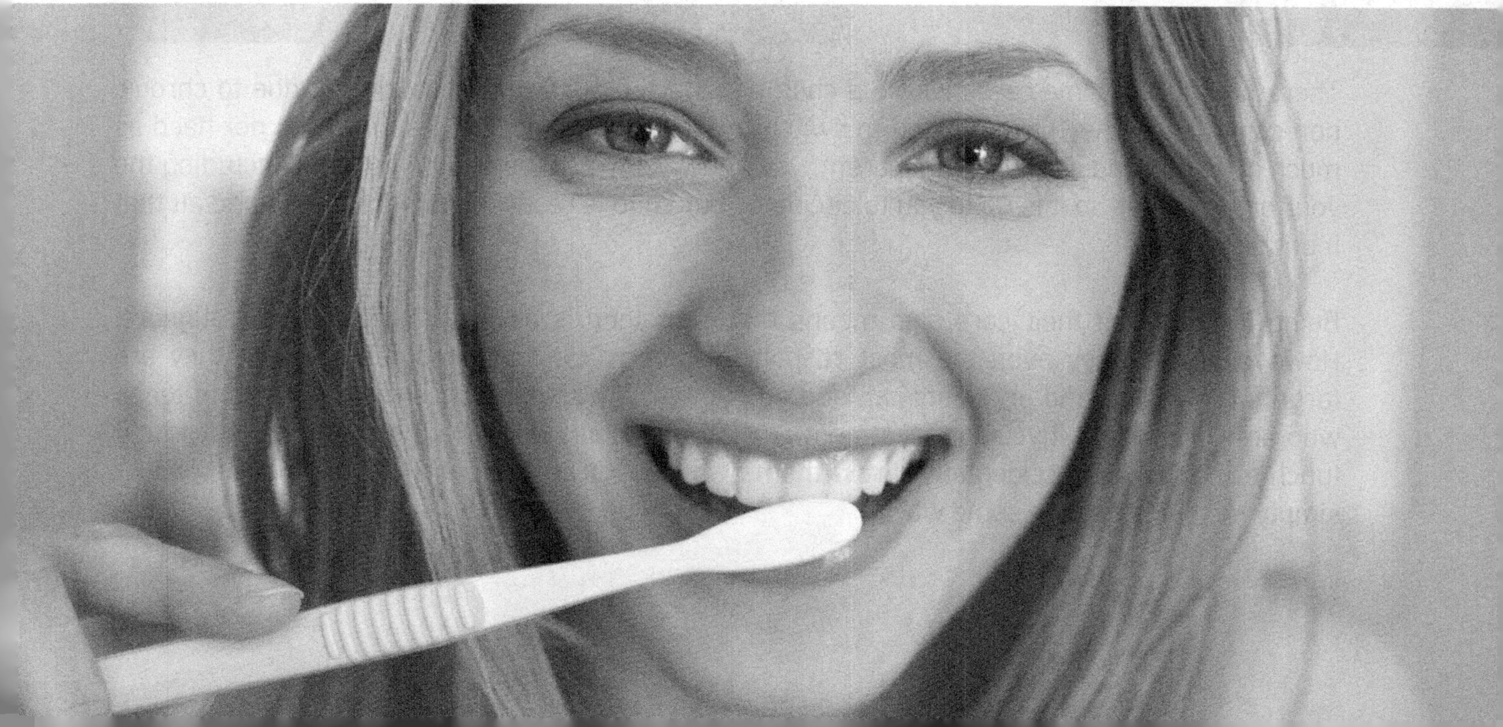

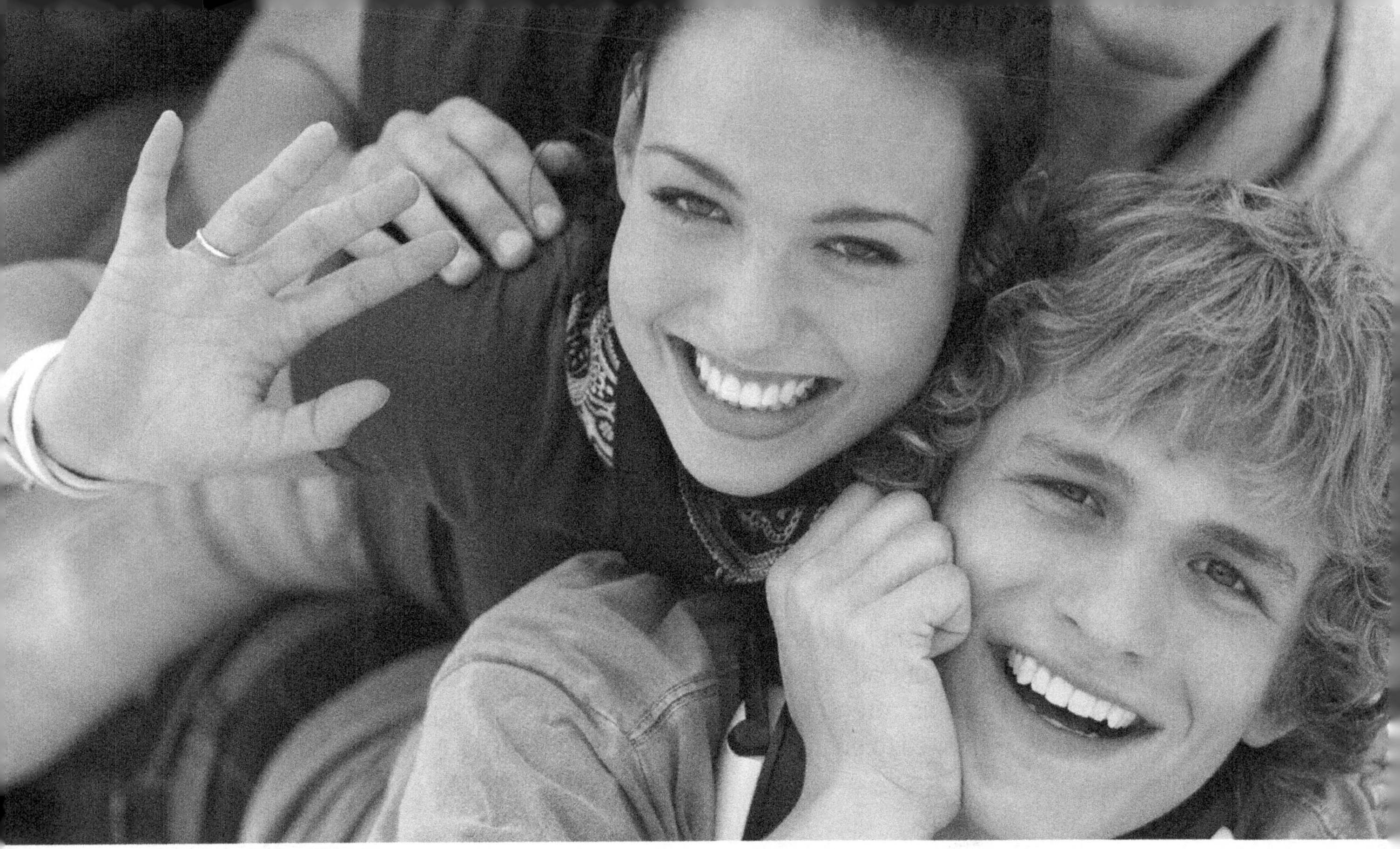

There have been some cases where a child has started out with Invisalign but due to chronic non-compliance, they have needed to switch to traditional metal braces which do not need as much attention and care. As their parent, you know your child better than anyone including the your orthodontist, so it is up to you to decide if your child is ready for this treatment and all that it entails.

Being in charge of their care also means that your teen is also in charge of their aligners. However, sometimes even the most responsible teens can have moments where they are forgetful. Mistakes and accidents can and do happen. A frequent concern for parents of teens who are undergoing Invisalign treatment is that their child will take their aligners out to eat lunch at school and accidentally throw them away, or leave them at a friend's house, or just simply misplace them in some way.

If your teen misplaces an aligner, you can simply contact your doctor's office and you will be given a new tray. The Invisalign Teen treatment plan provides you up to six complementary replacements. Depending on how close to the next set of aligners your teen is, they may be given a lateral replacement for their tray which is at their current stage, or just move on to the next set and not worry about getting a replacement.

Another important question that many parents ask, especially if they have not had the process of straightening their teeth done themselves, is this: does Invisalign hurt? The answer is that while aligners may feel a little uncomfortable at first, and for the first day or two that aligners are in for the first time, your child may have some difficulty speaking normally. This is temporary, however, and after a very short period (sometimes as short as a week), there should be no side effects and no pain from wearing the aligners.

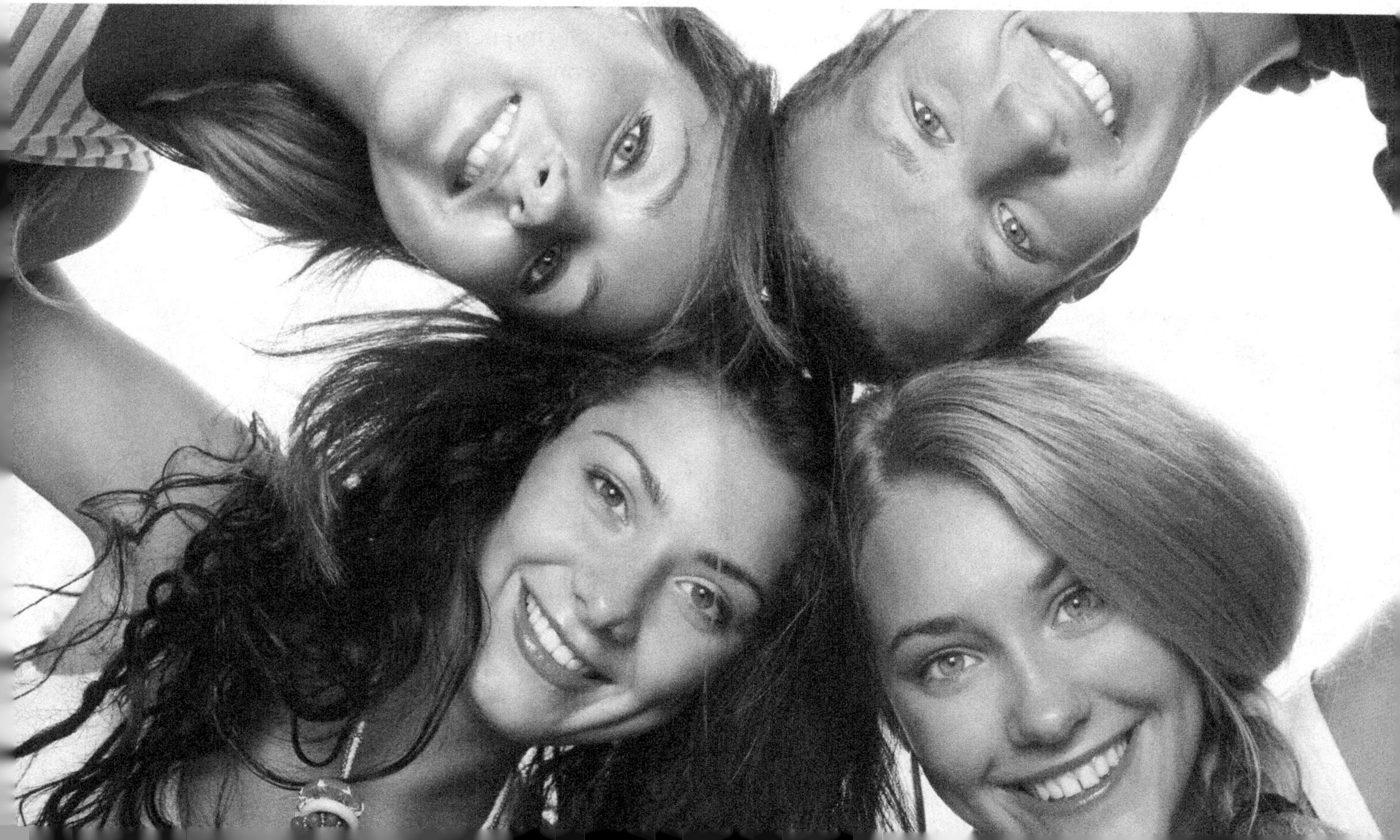

Having a child who wears braces also means you will have many appointments at your orthodontist's office. Invisalign offers benefits in this area as well, as it is a faster process to straighten your child's teeth. The typical treatment can take anywhere from 12-18 months, though in some cases it is shorter as it depends on the degree of straightening that needs to occur.

Since the overall process of treatment is faster, there are also far less visits involved in the process of straightening teeth with Invisalign. With changes to your teen's teeth being incremental and taking place over time, appointments are basically utilized to "check in" with your child to make sure that the corrections are progressing as they should.

Invisalign also eliminates the needs for emergency visits because your teen broke a wire or a bracket, or needs to have a wire tightened. This benefit is one that both parents and teens appreciate, and it removes the fear that any of these situations can occur when doing everyday life things, or that your teen will have a broken bracket during something like a family vacation where you aren't easily able to get to the orthodontist's office.

All of these previously mentioned benefits add up to provide one very important combined benefit: overall more efficient treatment.

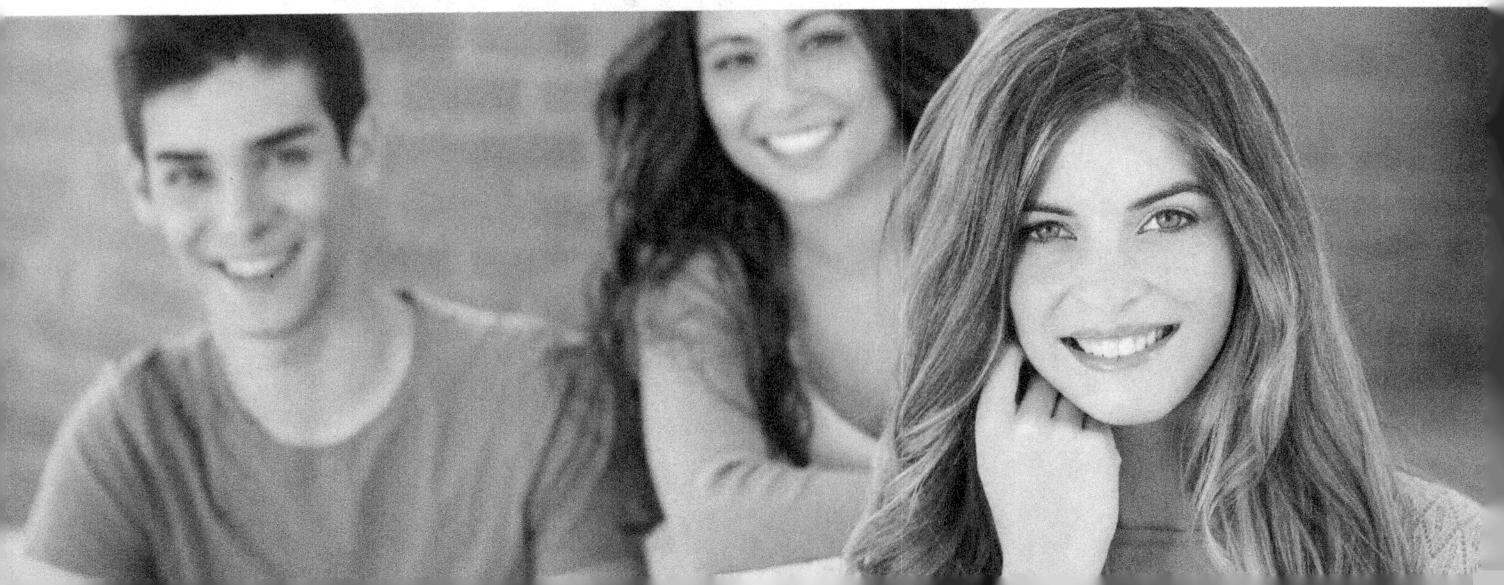

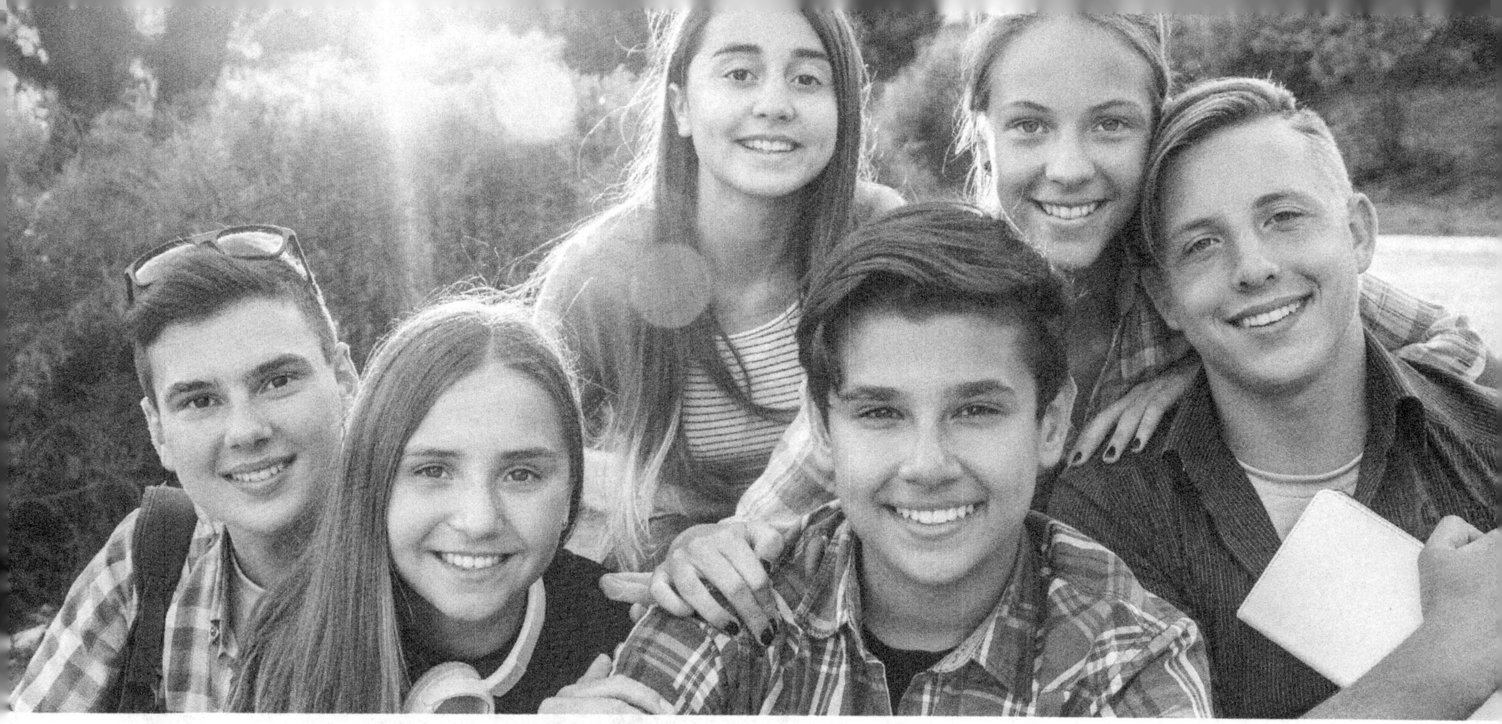

A very common misconception - and one which makes many parents decide on metal braces for their teens instead of Invisalign - is that Invisalign is going to be significantly more expensive. The truth is: that is not the case for most patients. While Invisalign's cost was higher than metal braces when it was a newly introduced method of treatment years ago, today the two methods cost roughly around the same amount.

Pricing varies by the degree of treatment that the teen may need, and there are other factors to consider as well, such as geographic location. Your doctor can discuss these things, along with payment plans, during your consultation.

With the numerous benefits that Invisalign offers as a way to correct issues such as over/ underbite, gapped or crooked teeth, it is easy to see why it is such a popular option with both parents and teens.

You may not have an option as to whether or not your child needs braces, but this "clear" alternative will definitely ease some of your teen's (and your) anxiety about the process.

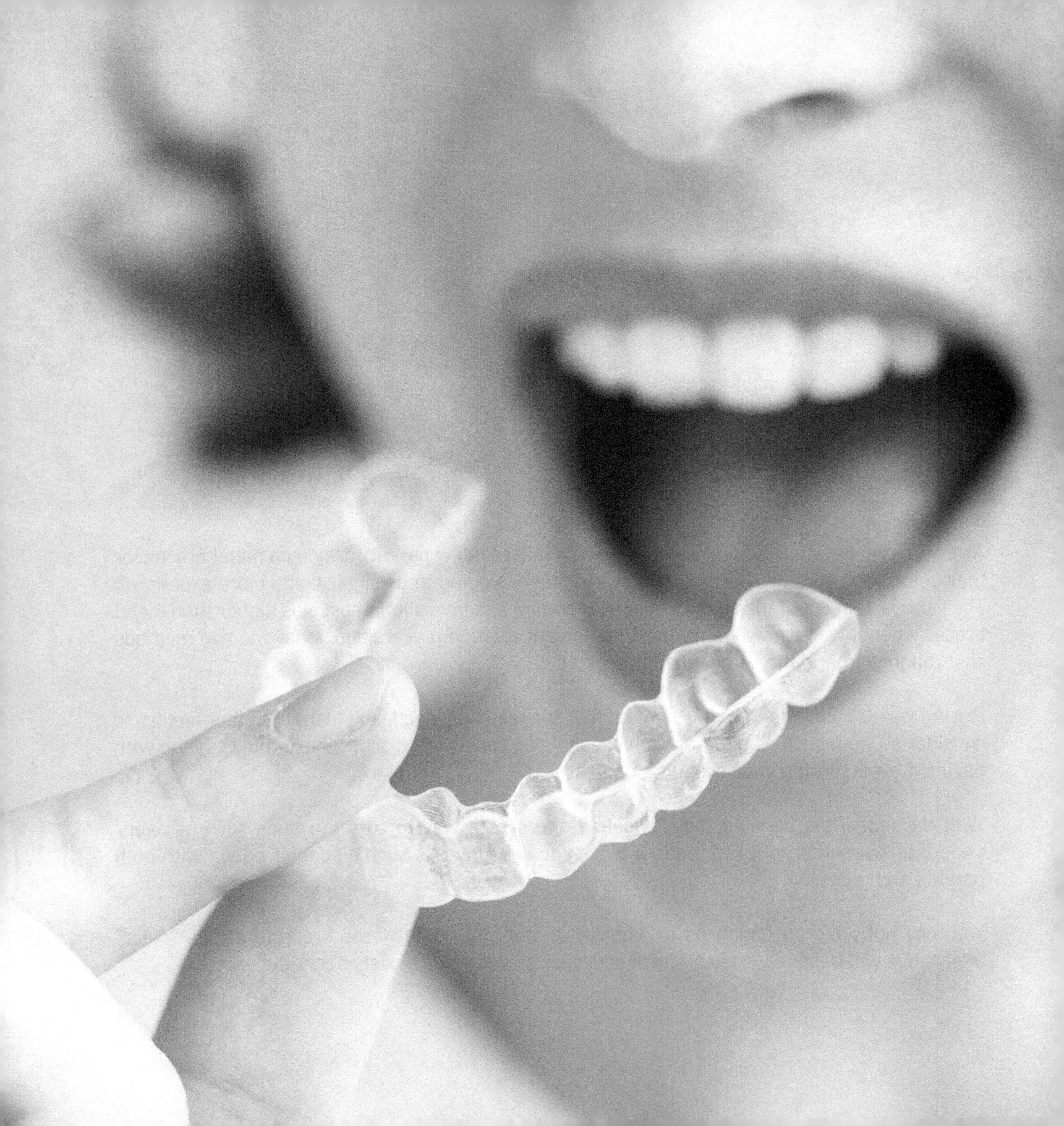

Treatment for Adults

It is pretty well known that most orthodontists recommend straightening your teeth during your teenage years. This is mainly because a person's teeth are easier to move until around age twenty, so when correction is done before that age, the process tends to be more efficient than when you are older.

This doesn't mean that anyone over the age of twenty is resigned to living with crooked teeth - far from it! If you have been considering getting braces because you were unable to do so at a young age (either for financial reasons or otherwise) - it is not too late! People are living longer now than ever before, and a growing number of adults have been opting to seek orthodontic treatment. It is estimated that approximately 20-30% of people who wear braces are adults.

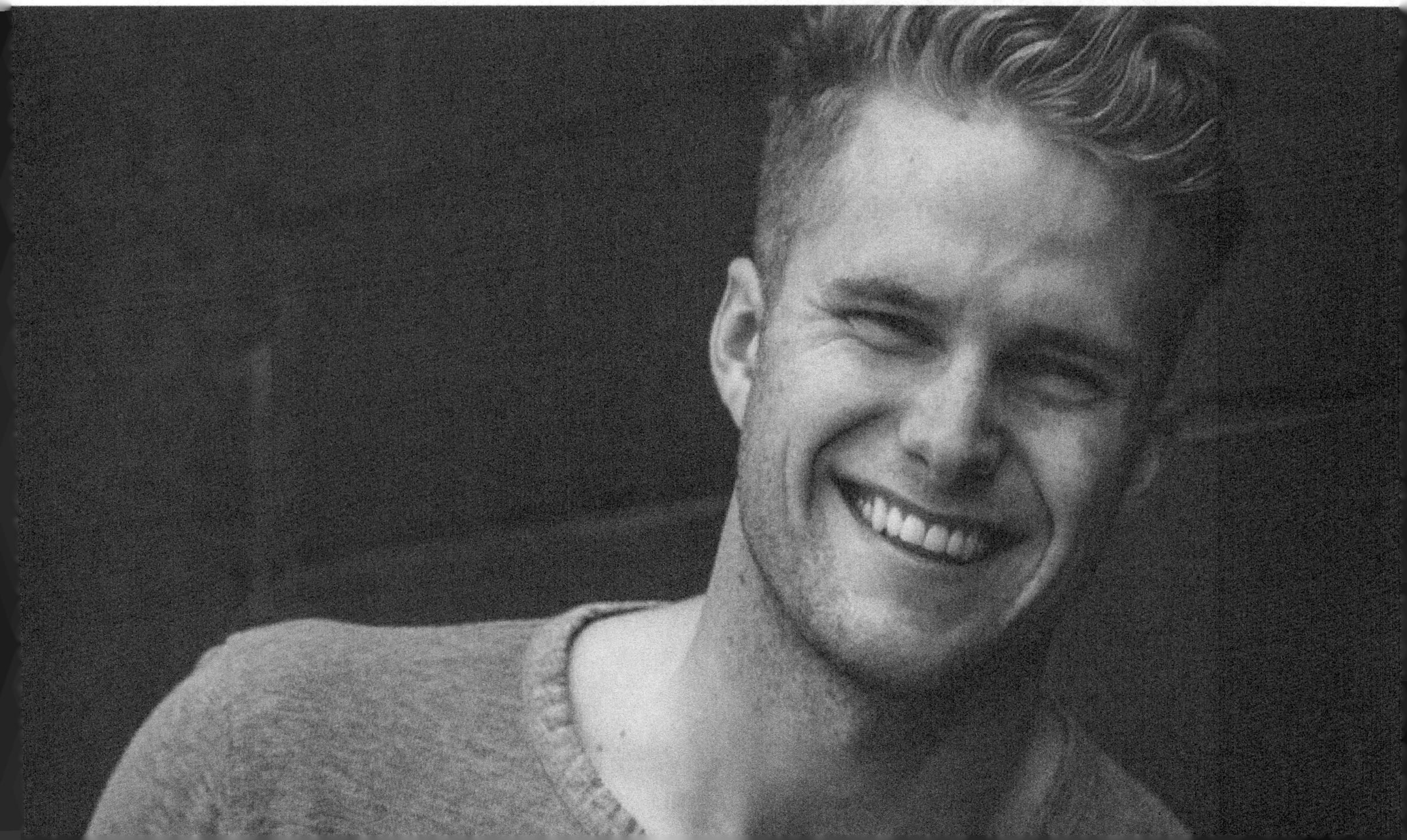

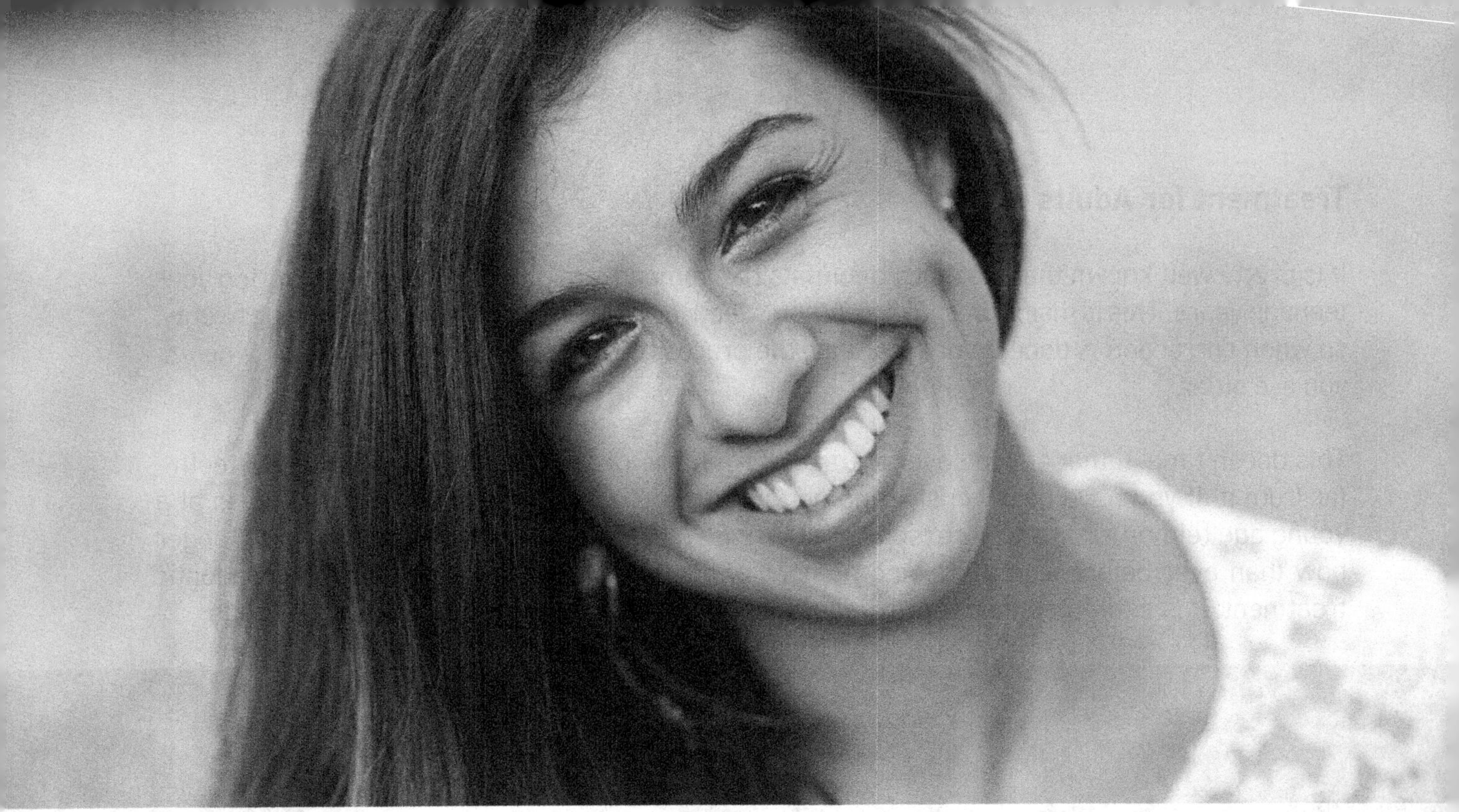

Research has proven time and again that smiling is directly linked to your self confidence and it increases your happiness in life. It is a great way to lift not just your own mood but that of others around you as well. One reason is because smiling releases neurotransmitters called endorphins - which lowers your stress level, relaxes your body, and lowers your blood pressure and heart rate.

Your smile affects how others perceive you, and most people agree that it makes you more attractive and friendly looking. When you smile at another person, you are expressing to them that you like them and find them pleasant in your estimation. That simple act is so powerful that it can often jolt a person with low esteem from negativity into positivity. Smiles have even been the catalyst of countless numbers of relationships and even marriages - many people report that they first noticed and then became interested in their significant other after sharing a smile across a room.

The bottom line is that every time you smile, you not only make other people feel better about themselves, but you get many benefits too.

If you already have a great smile, chances are you don't think about it much - you just smile. However, when you have unattractive or crooked teeth, you are more inclined to hide your smile than you are to show it to others - despite all of the many benefits you gain from doing so.

Many people feel that having unattractive or crooked teeth holds them back from achievement and living their most fulfilling life. While there is not one "magic bullet" that dictates what makes a person successful or motivates them to meet their potential, it is clear that self esteem and confidence are two traits that all successful people have. And it has been proven that smiling ranks highly among simple things that you can do to boost both characteristics.

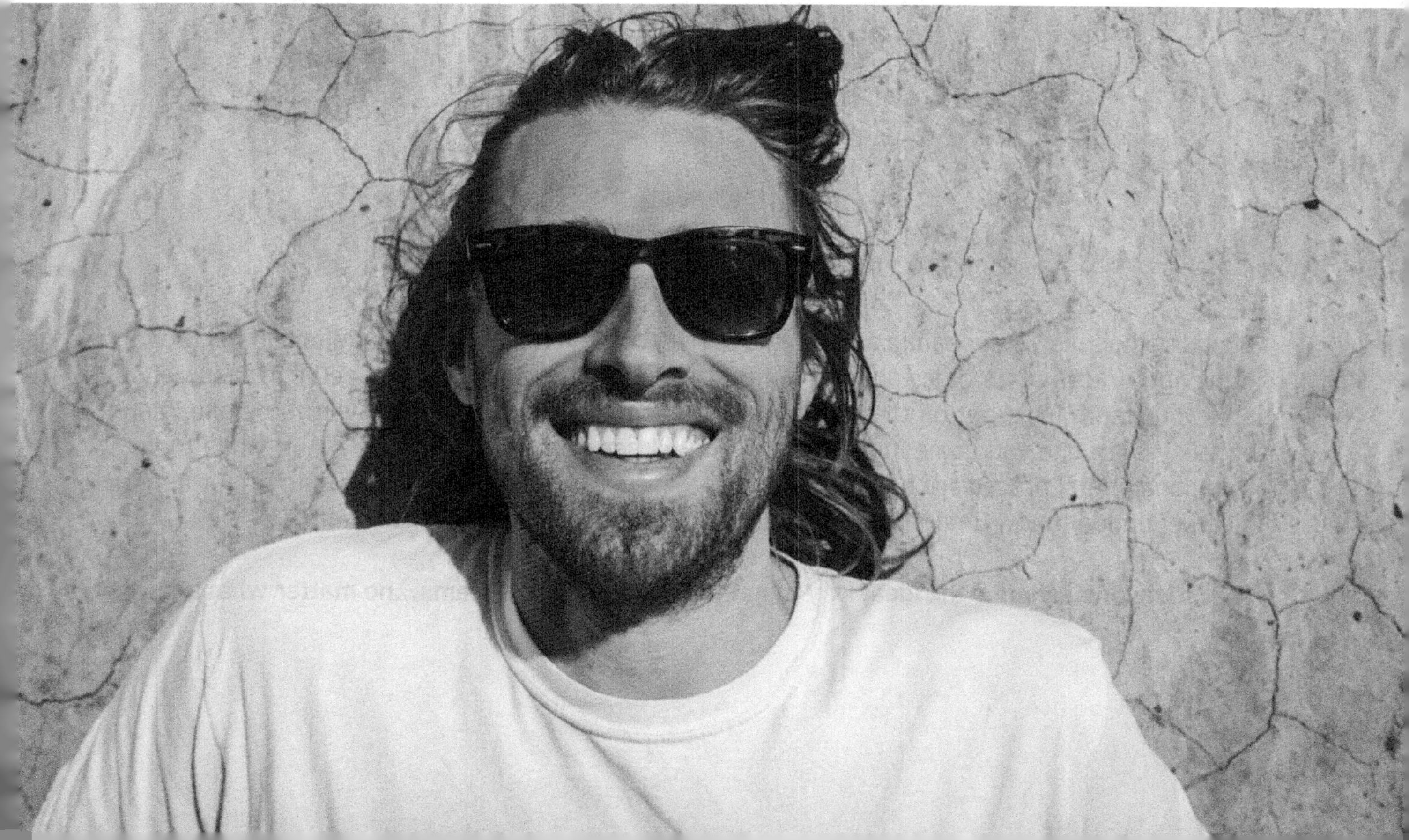

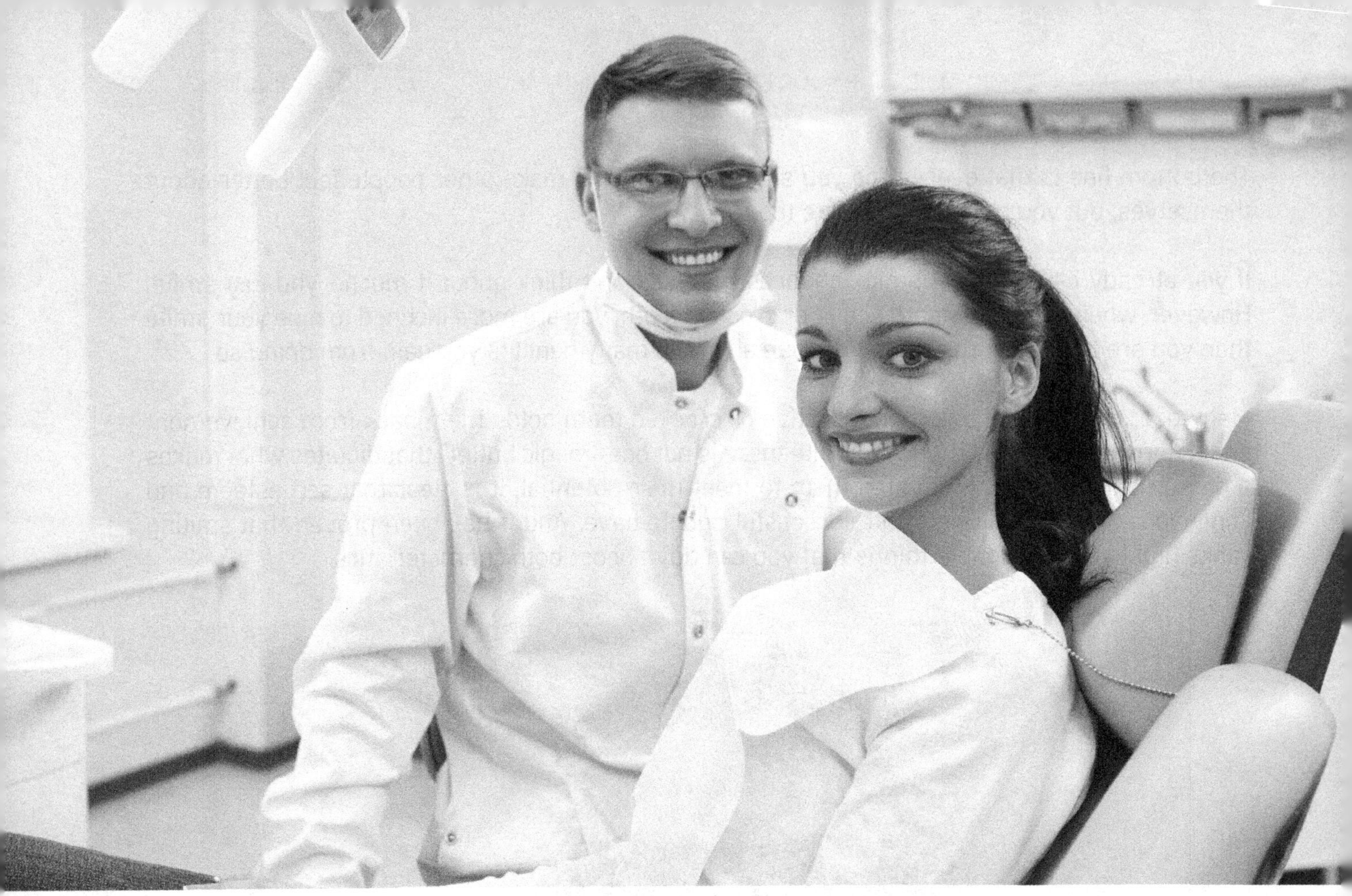

Despite all of this, as appealing as having a "perfect" smile may be, many adults find the thought of having braces at an older age very off-putting. On one hand, you may self-conscious about how your teeth look, but on the other - you are keenly aware that whenever you smile, laugh or talk - everyone you come into contact with will see you wearing braces. And while today's traditional metal braces are better than they have ever been - most adults would prefer a more discreet option that will not make them further self-conscious about their teeth.

That's why Invisalign is the ideal way to get the smile of your dreams...no matter what age you are!

Invisalign for adults work much like Invisalign Teen works, which we discussed earlier in this book. You will be provided a series of trays that work to incrementally move your teeth into position, and this process will continue until you achieve your desired results. Invisalign treatment for adults can take an average of 12-18 months, but like with the teen version, this is wholly dependent on the severity of the correction that needs to be made. You also need to make sure that you follow the treatment plan that is given to you by your doctor, and that you follow the suggested wear of your aligners of approximately 22 hours per day for maximum effectiveness.

As we have previously discussed in earlier sections, there are not dietary restrictions for patients who wear Invisalign as you must remove your aligners before eating or drinking anything other than water. You should also make sure to keep up with your regular brushing and flossing habits as well.

It is important to note that even if you have had braces as a child, teeth can move at any age – including well into adulthood. And when they do, they can affect not just the aesthetics of your smile but many other unseen issues.

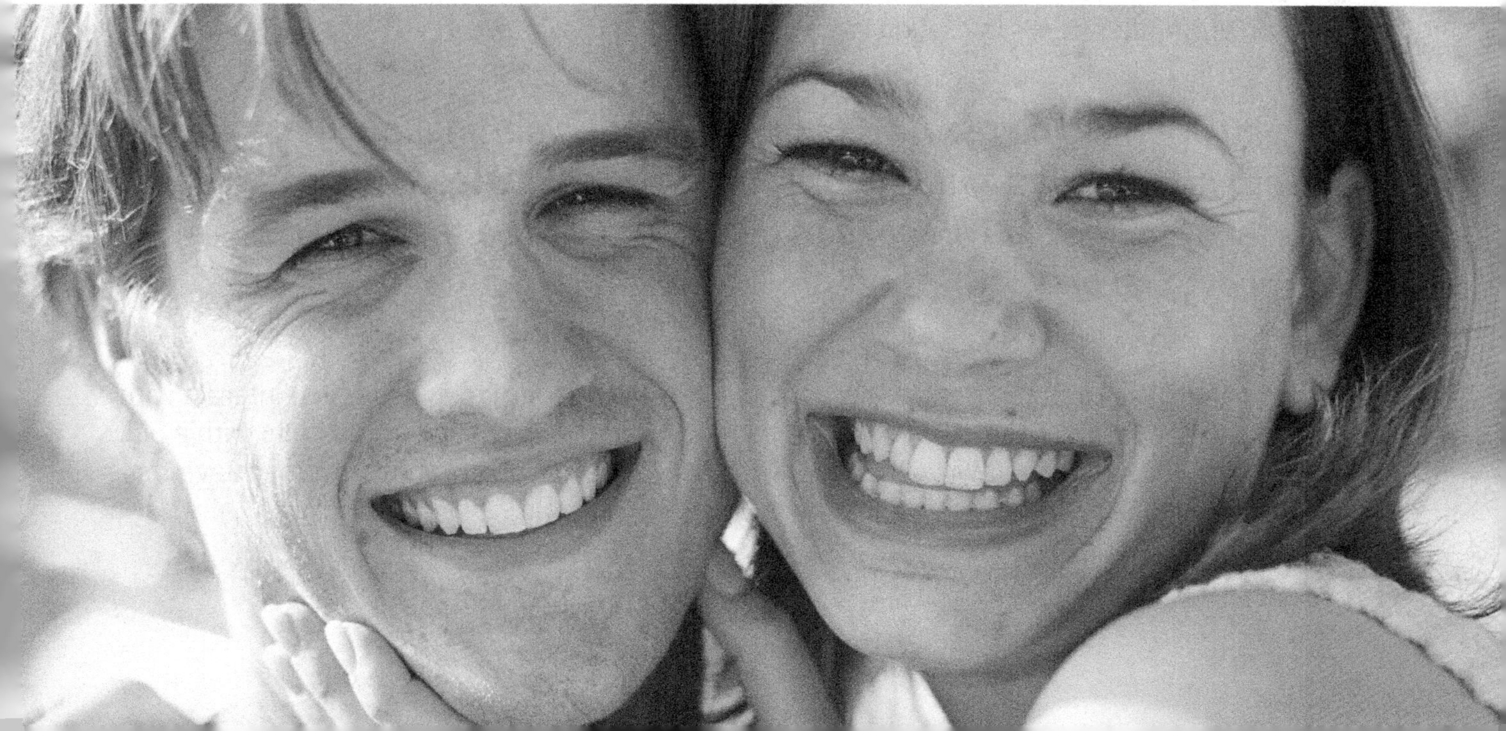

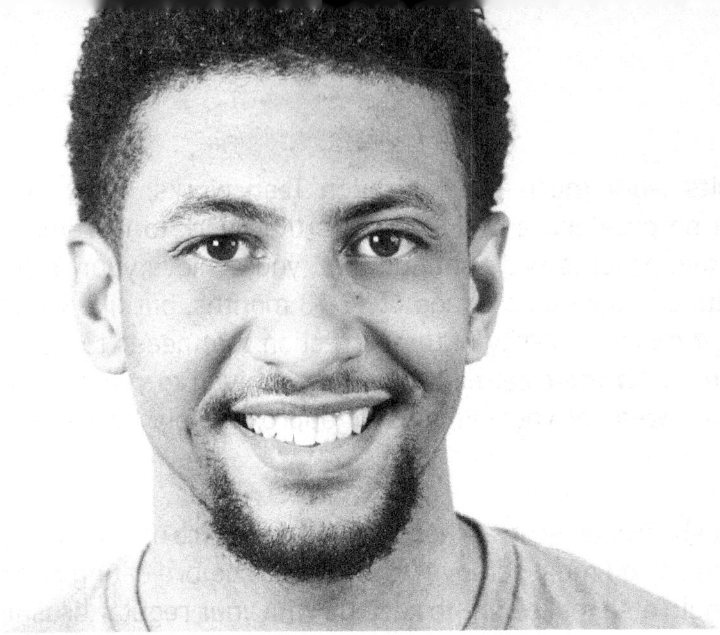

Crooked or misaligned teeth can cause jaw pain, create difficulty in proper cleaning routines, and even cause gastrointestinal problems from not chewing your food properly. Other more serious issues such as missing/broken teeth can also cause shifting issues that put you at risk for all of these aforementioned issues as well as other long term discomforts such as headaches, neck and back pain. These factors are also things you should consider when you are making the decision of whether or not Invisalign is right for you.

If you are missing teeth and are considering getting implants, your teeth must be straight first. If you have crooked teeth in addition to missing teeth, you will need to get braces before the implant process can begin.

Having healthy, straight teeth will make a huge difference in your life and how you interact with others. Say goodbye to being self-conscious about your smile...and instead say hello with a big, beautiful smile that you will want to share with everyone. Invisalign can help you achieve that goal in a reasonable amount of time...with truly amazing results!

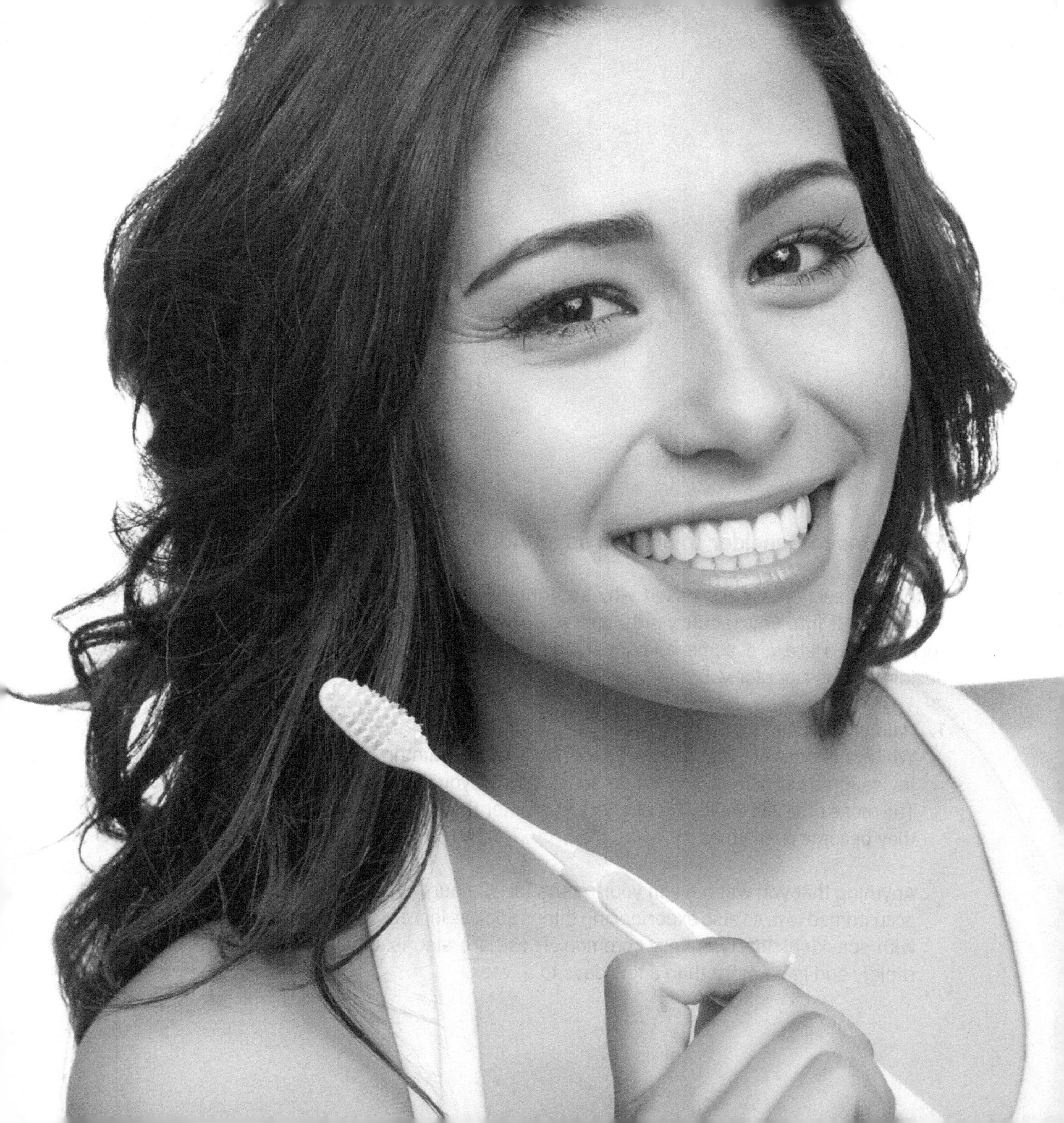

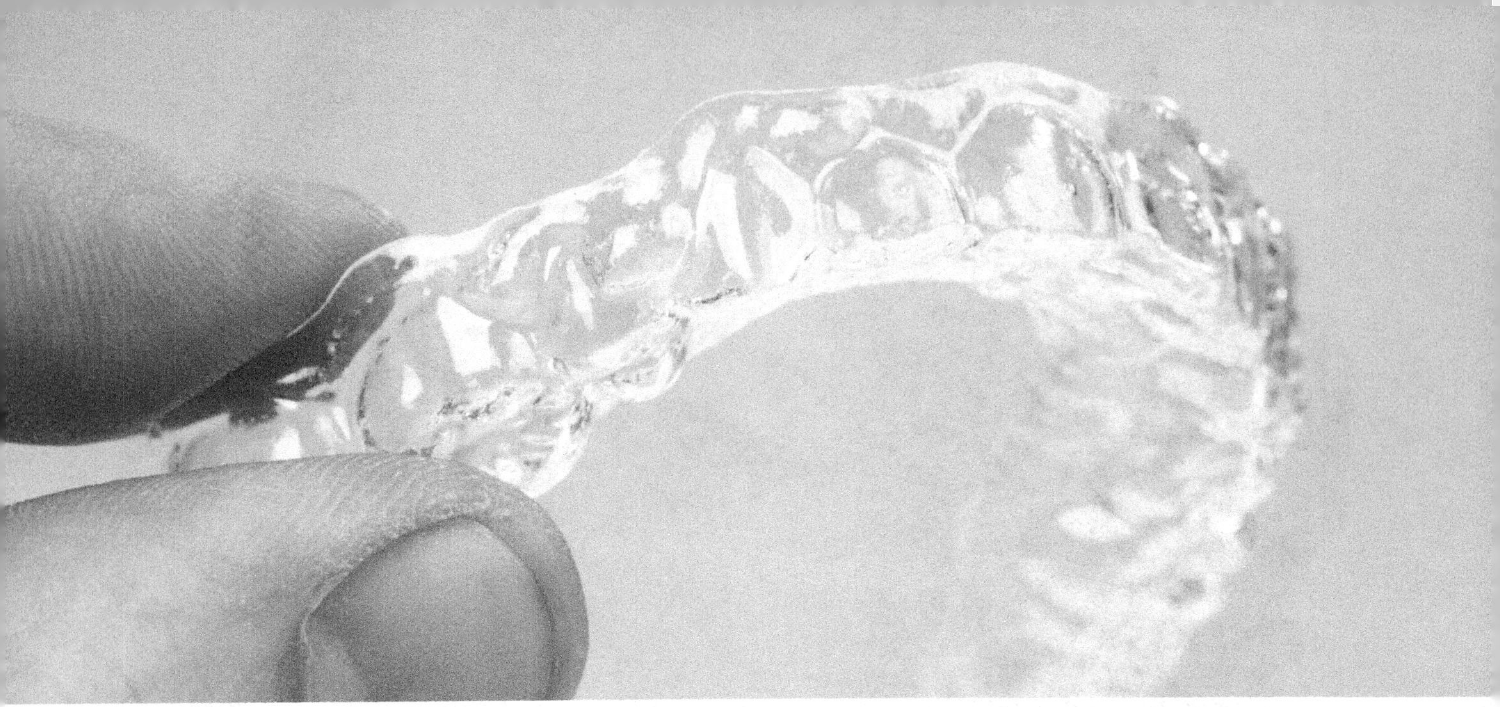

5 Reasons to Consider Invisalign as an Adult

In the last section, we discussed why straightening your teeth is a good decision even when you are well into your adult years, and why Invisalign may be a good choice to make those corrections. Here are some additional points about Invisalign treatment to consider when deciding if it is right for you.

1. **Pain is minimal.**
   While it is possible that you will experience some pain or discomfort when you begin your Invisalign treatment, it will not be an issue after you being wearing your aligners regularly. The more time you wear your aligners, the faster they tend to adjust and the more comfortable they become over time.

   Anything that you will have in your mouth for 22 hours is going to require your mouth to get accustomed to it, so also experiencing things such as increased saliva production and difficulty with speaking clearly is very common. These are also issues that will correct themselves rapidly and in no more than a few days to a week.

2. **Treatment does not last forever - but a beautiful smile will.**
   One of the questions that we hear the most about getting treatment is: "How long is this going to take?" There is no definitive answer as treatment time varies by patient. However, something to keep in mind that the time you spend in treatment - including the time after you are done with your aligner trays and are wearing a retainer - is relatively short by comparison to the rest of your life. When you complete treatment successfully, your result is a beautiful and healthy smile that will last you a lifetime. Anyone can see that a little investment of time to improve your smile, your health and in turn, your life - is time that is well spent.

3. **Treatment time may be less than you expect.**
   Choosing Invisalign as your treatment option to straighten your teeth takes, on average, twelve to eighteen months to obtain your desired results. There are also cases where a patient's correction happens faster than the average time frame It is impossible to predict an exact time that a patient will be in treatment, but overall it is generally a faster period than traditional braces.

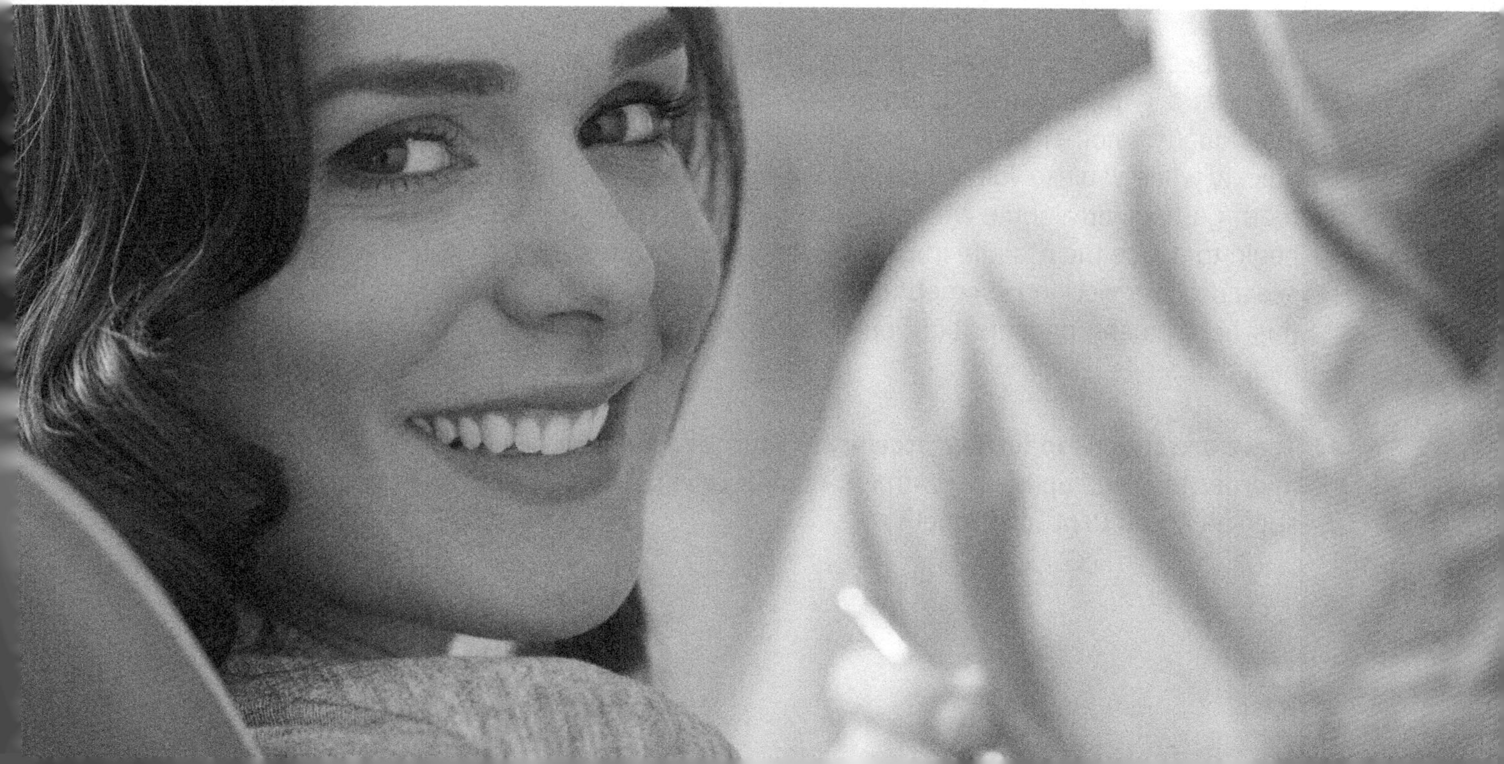

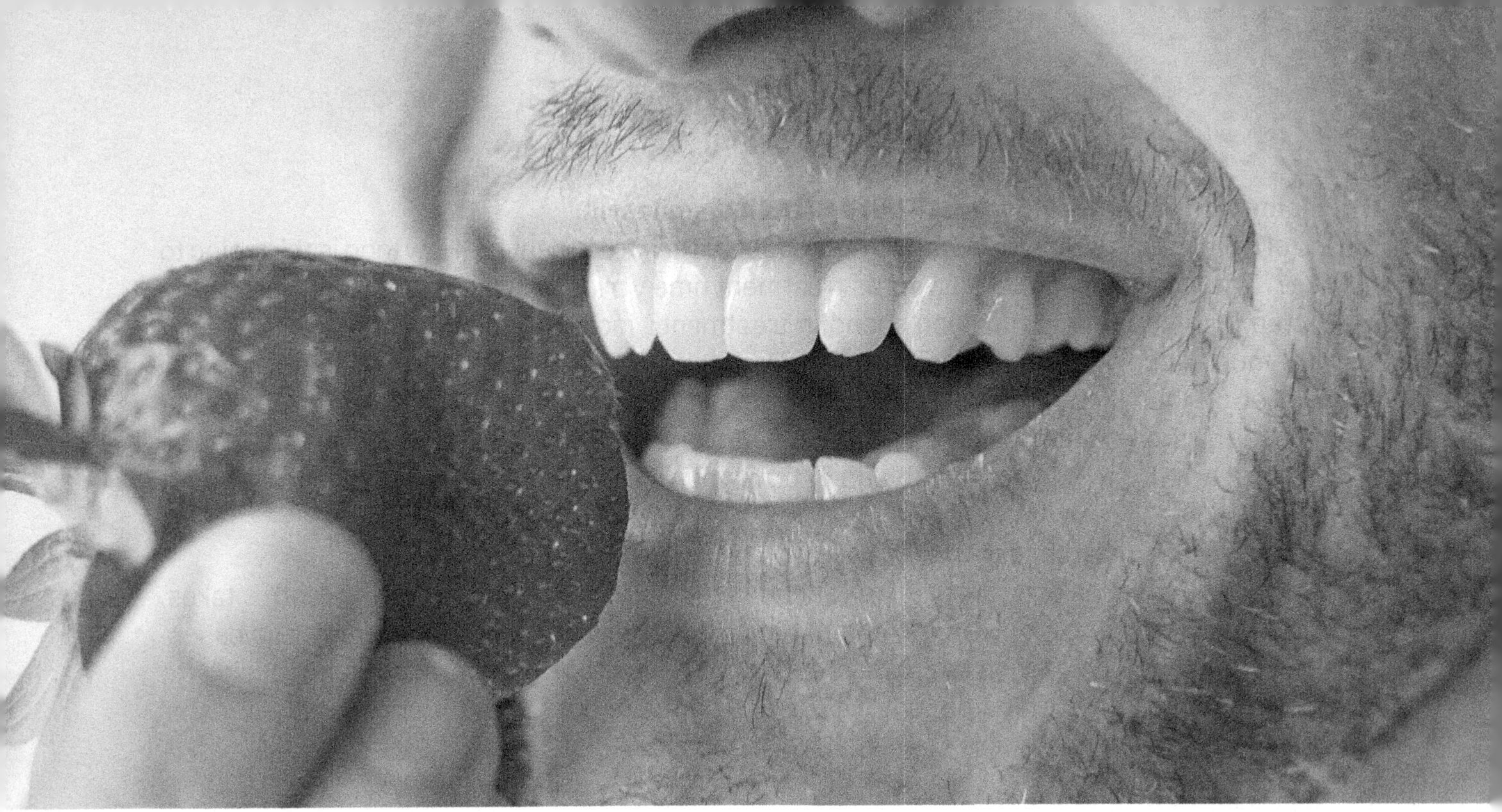

This is because your Invisalign aligners use a different process to move your teeth - it moves them as a whole. This is different than how metal braces work, which move each tooth individually. Another benefit of Invisalign treatment is that you start to notice results relatively quickly when you use your aligners as directed. Most patients begin to see changes and their teeth getting straighter within two to three months, and they have reported that others begin to notice their smile improvements a few months after that. It is a great motivator to see a process working - something that is far more difficult to do with traditional braces - and this helps many patients stay on track and focused on their goal of a perfectly straight, beautiful smile.

4. **There are options to further accelerate your treatment.**
   In order to speed up their treatment times, some patients opt to use additional procedures such as AcceleDent® or Propel®.

AcceleDent is an FDA approved appliances which you can use at home for approximately 20 minutes a day. It uses micro-pulse technology to speed up the movement of your teeth. This not only cuts your treatment time with Invisalign much shorter, but it also gently massages your teeth which many patients report soothes the discomfort of wearing a new aligner tray whenever their old one is switched out.

Propel is a treatment that is done in your doctor's office. It works by stimulating bone remodeling, allowing your teeth to straighten faster when it works in conjunction with your Invisalign aligners. When starting the process, your doctor takes x-rays and determines the ideal spot in your jaw to make a series of small holes, called micro-osteoperforations. These holes help to make the bone more pliable on both sides of your tooth, making it easier to relocate it to it's proper spot.

Patients report that treatment with Propel feels similar to having a deep cleaning done by a dental hygienist. The process is virtually painless and only takes a few minutes to complete.

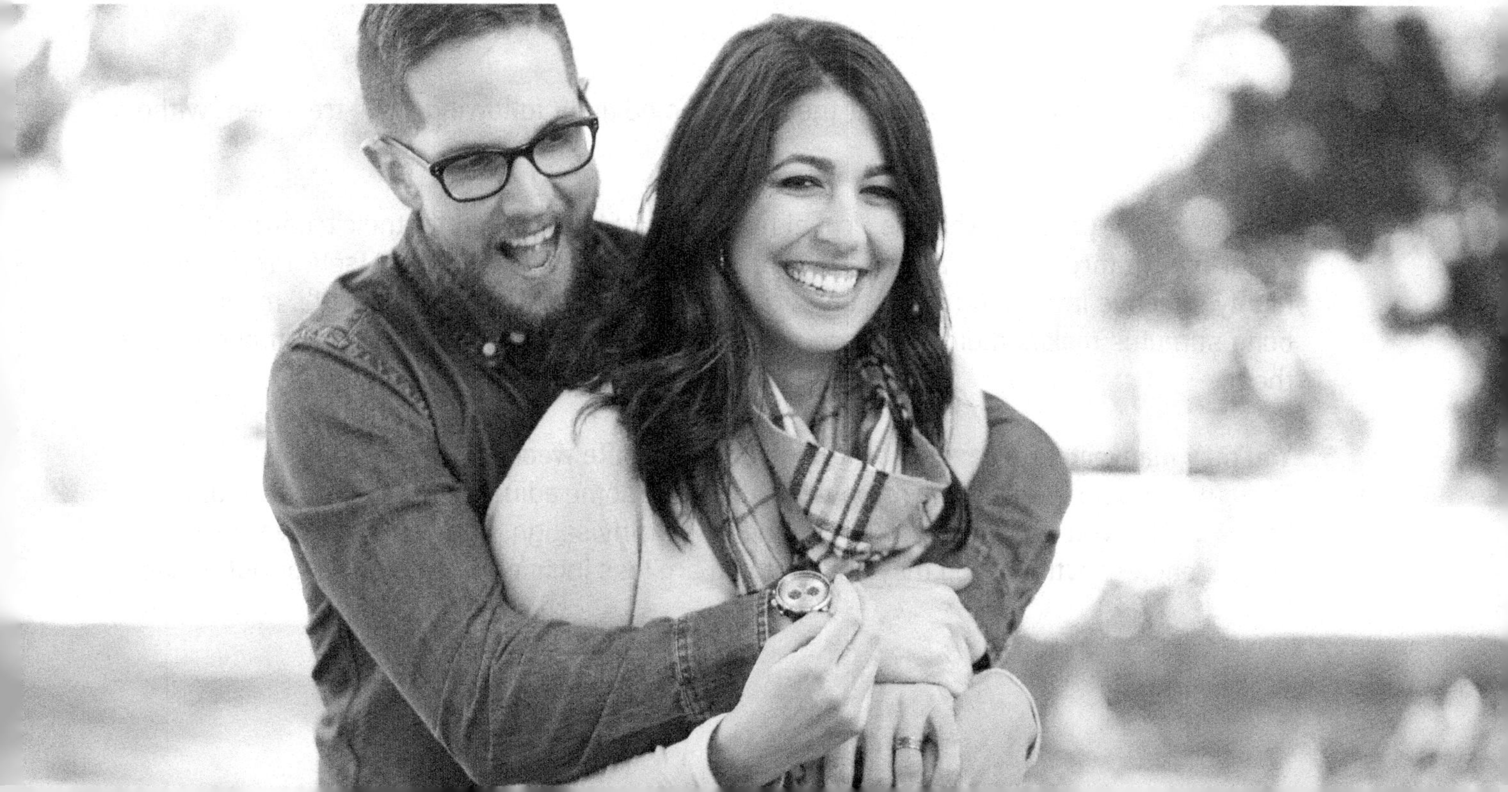

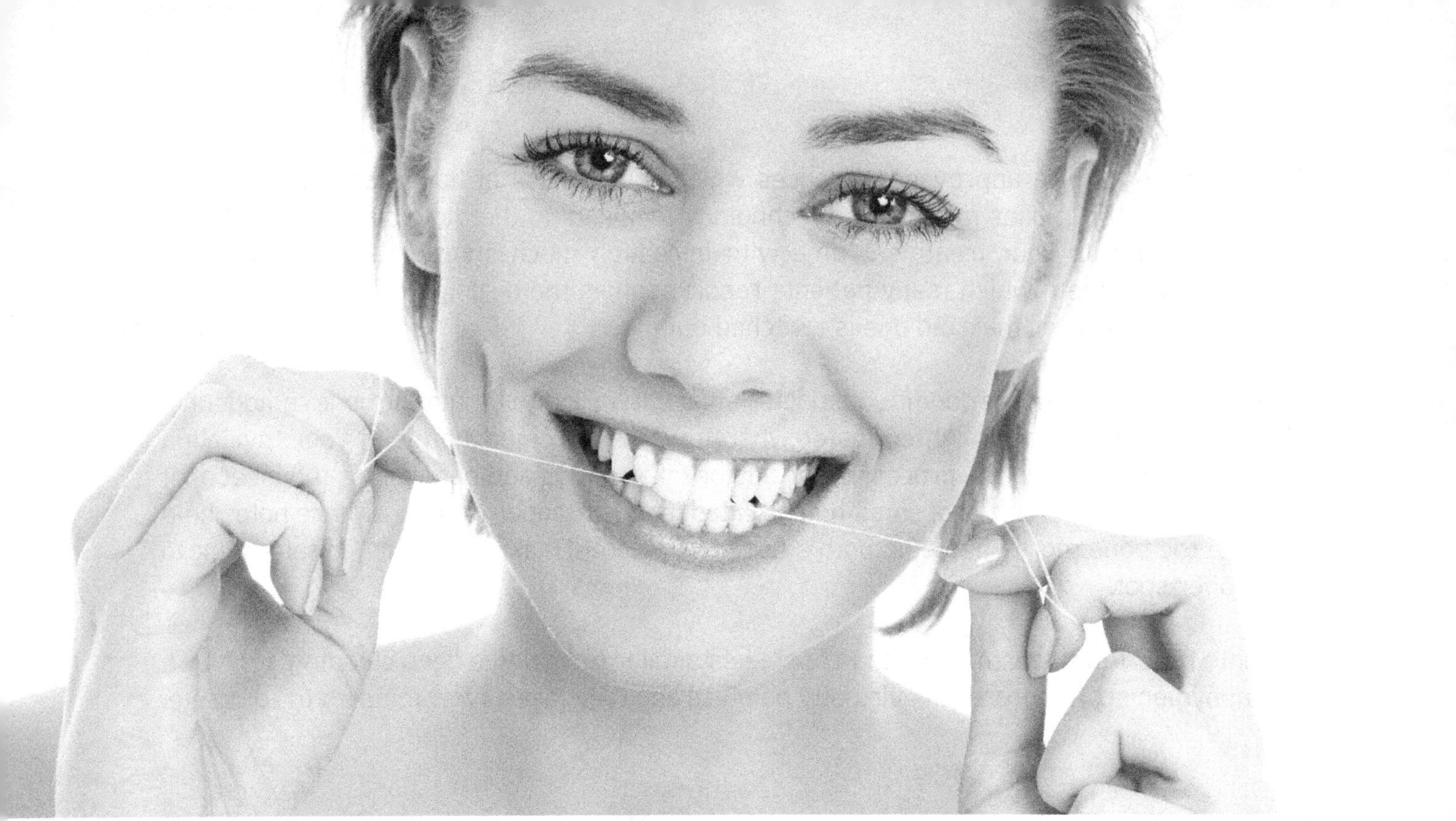

Most patients are able to go about their day immediately following their treatment without any impact.

In many cases, patients who use Propel have been able to complete their treatment times about two to three times faster than those who opt for Invisalign by itself. Propel is also highly effective in treating more complicated cases of crowding in a patient's mouth as the bone stimulus makes their jaw more adaptive to the shifting of the teeth with aligners on them.

5. **You may inadvertently develop other good habits while wearing Invisalign.**
Even though your aligners are removable, there are some adjustments to make to your eating habits while you are undergoing treatment with Invisalign. You must remove your trays before eating anything, you may find that you are less inclined to eat snacks or out of habit

versus actual hunger, because you are aware that you must brush your teeth following any food consumption, and before you place your aligners back in your mouth. Many patients report losing a few pounds while undergoing treatment, which they commonly refer to as "The InvisalignDiet".

Drinking anything other than water also requires you to repeat the process of removing your aligners, brushing and replacing as well. This causes many patients to substitute less healthy, sugary drinks like soda with water because it's easier. This is not a bad thing, as the benefits of drinking more water are well known. Drinking more water also helps keep your mouth from being dry or irritated when wearing your aligners.

Many Invisalign patients also find that having the treatment with aligners improves their existing oral hygiene habits. The removable nature of your aligners makes it so that you brush your teeth often - most likely more often than you may have before starting the treatment. Better brushing and flossing habits are always a plus and help to improve your overall health. After completing a treatment such as Invisalign, you will left with a beautiful, healthy, straight smile - and you will want to keep it that way! Keeping up good brushing and flossing habits you developed during treatment are a great way to achieve this.

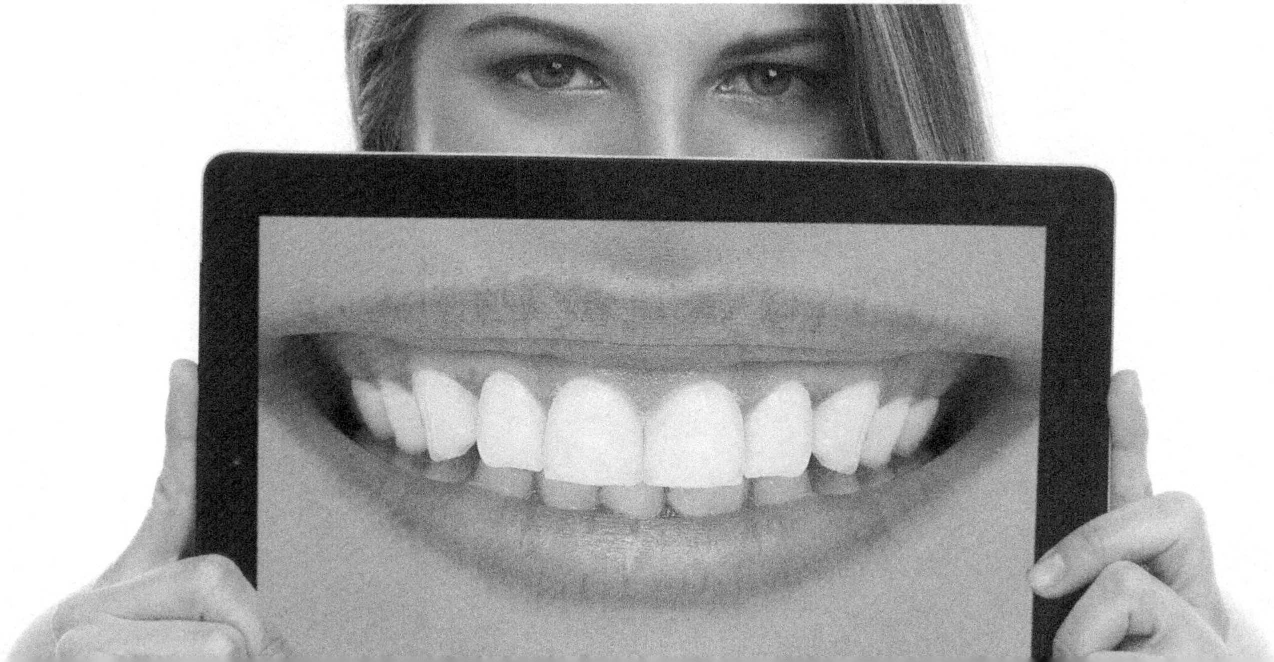

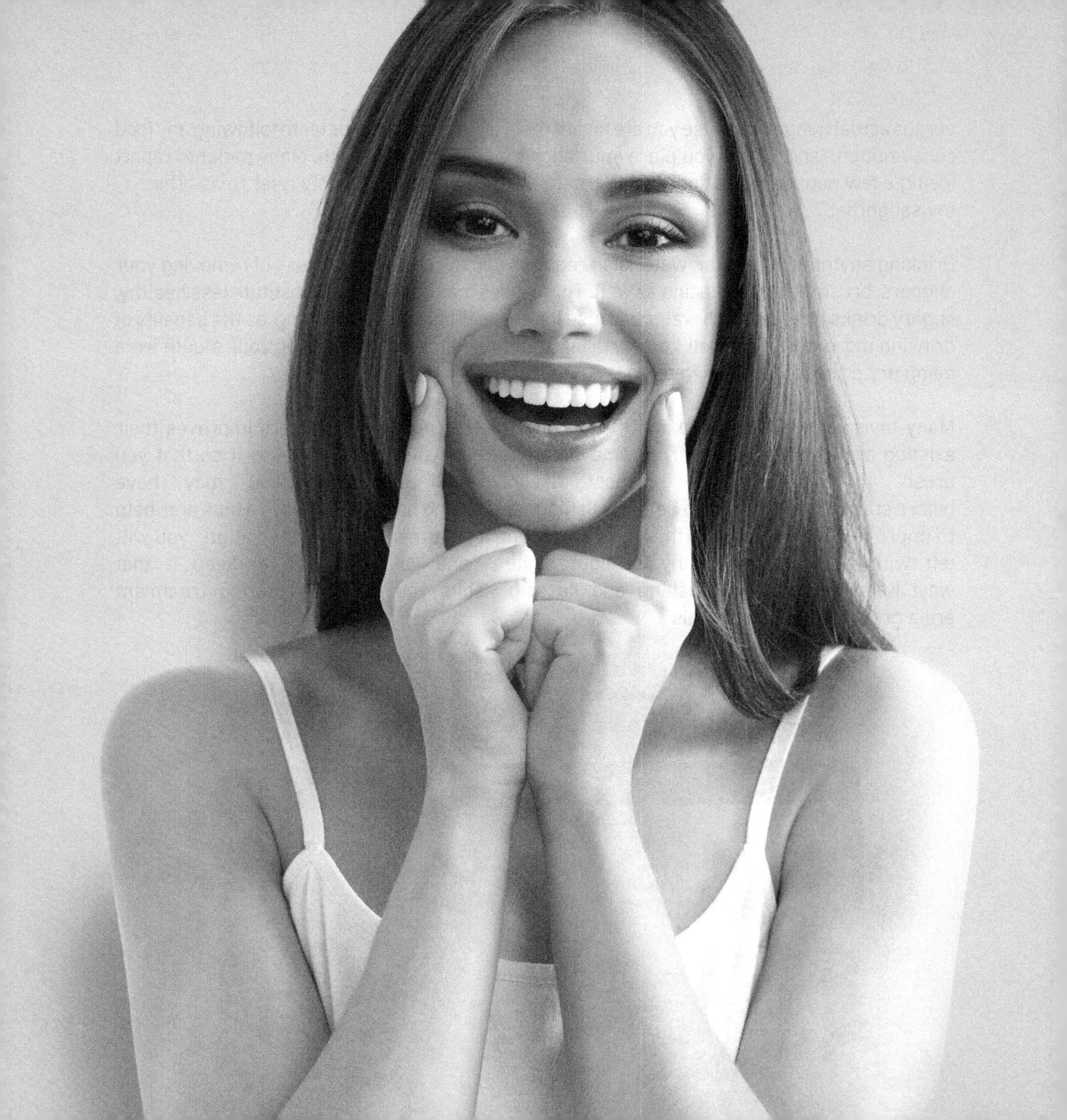

Chapter 2: How Invisalign Works

Invisalign aligners are made out of a patented thermoplastic material called SmartTrack®, which was formulated exclusively for use with Invisalign. The material is a flexible plastic which is FDA approved and contains no metal, BPAs, latex or gluten. They are thin and clear - making them virtually invisible.

The system works in a series of trays which gradually and incrementally shift your teeth into place so they are in a straight arrangement. Aligners are formulated so that they are slightly straighter than your teeth are, putting pressure on your teeth so that over the course of wear, your teeth will move to match the position of the aligner. Each aligner is approximately 0.25 millimeters straighter that the previous one in the series.

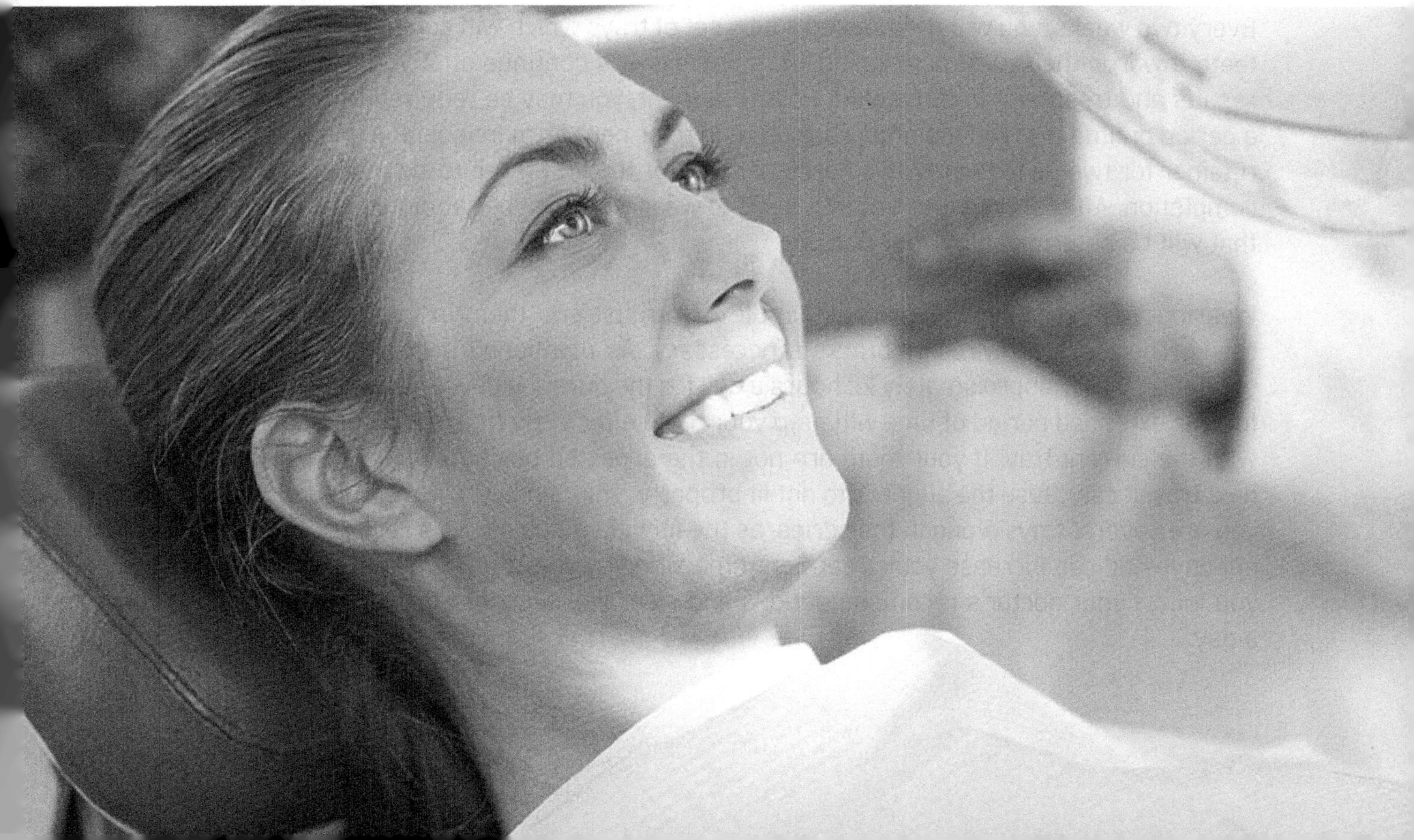

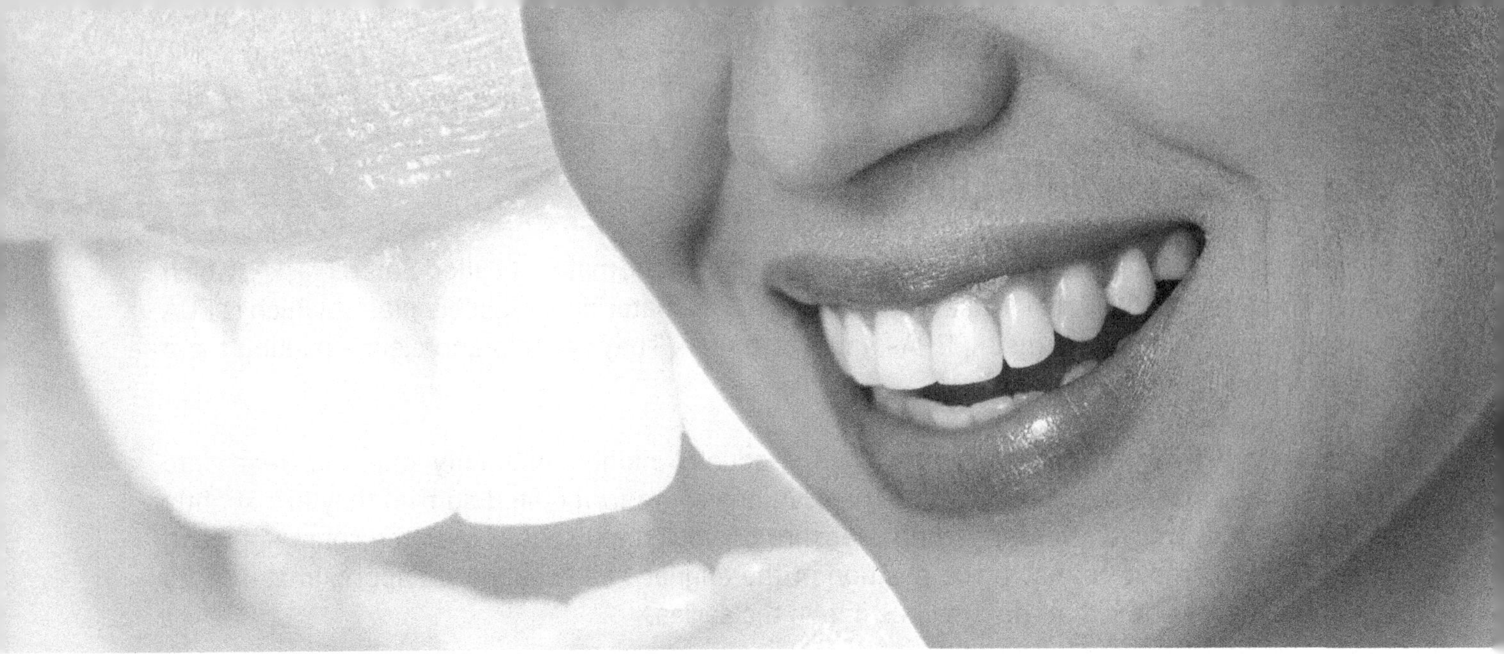

Every two weeks, you will be supplied a new set of trays which will continue slowly moving your teeth towards their ideal positioning. This process will continue until you achieve your desired results and treatment is completed. Post treatment, you may be required to wear a retainer for a period of time that will maintain your teeth in their new, straight position. Most patients wear a retainer for twelve to twenty-two hours per day for the first three to six months after treatment completion. After six months, you will need to wear your retainer at night time only for a period that will be determined by your doctor.

Wearing your Invisalign aligners is simple – you just pop them in your mouth and they are ready. There are no wires or brackets necessary. As mentioned previously, you should wear your aligners for approximately 22 hours a day for the duration of your treatment. Wearing them for this extended period of time will help your teeth effectively move into position in compliance with the current tray. If your teeth are not in the expected position when you move on to your next tray, it can cause the aligners to not fit properly. This can become a continued problem once you are several trays along in the series, as the fit will still be off. This renders the aligners less effective and can increase your treatment time significantly. That's why it's very important that you follow your doctor's recommendations and wear your aligners for the suggested 22 hours a day.

As your treatment progresses, you will need to visit your doctor's office approximately ever 6-8 weeks to make sure that your treatment is going smoothly and there are no issues which have arisen. Treatment times, as we have mentioned previously in this book, vary from patient to patient, but the average treatment period is 12-18 months. During this time, you can expect to wear anywhere from twenty to fifty trays, however, this number will also vary depending on the level of correction that is being done.

How Your Treatment Plan is Developed

The first step to getting started with Invisalign is a consultation with a dental professional who is an experienced Invisalign provider. During this assessment, your doctor will evaluate whether or not Invisalign is right for you, what issues you would like to have fixed, and what the severity of your case is. For cases where the correction needed is more complex, it may be necessary to have certain procedures done before you can begin treatment.

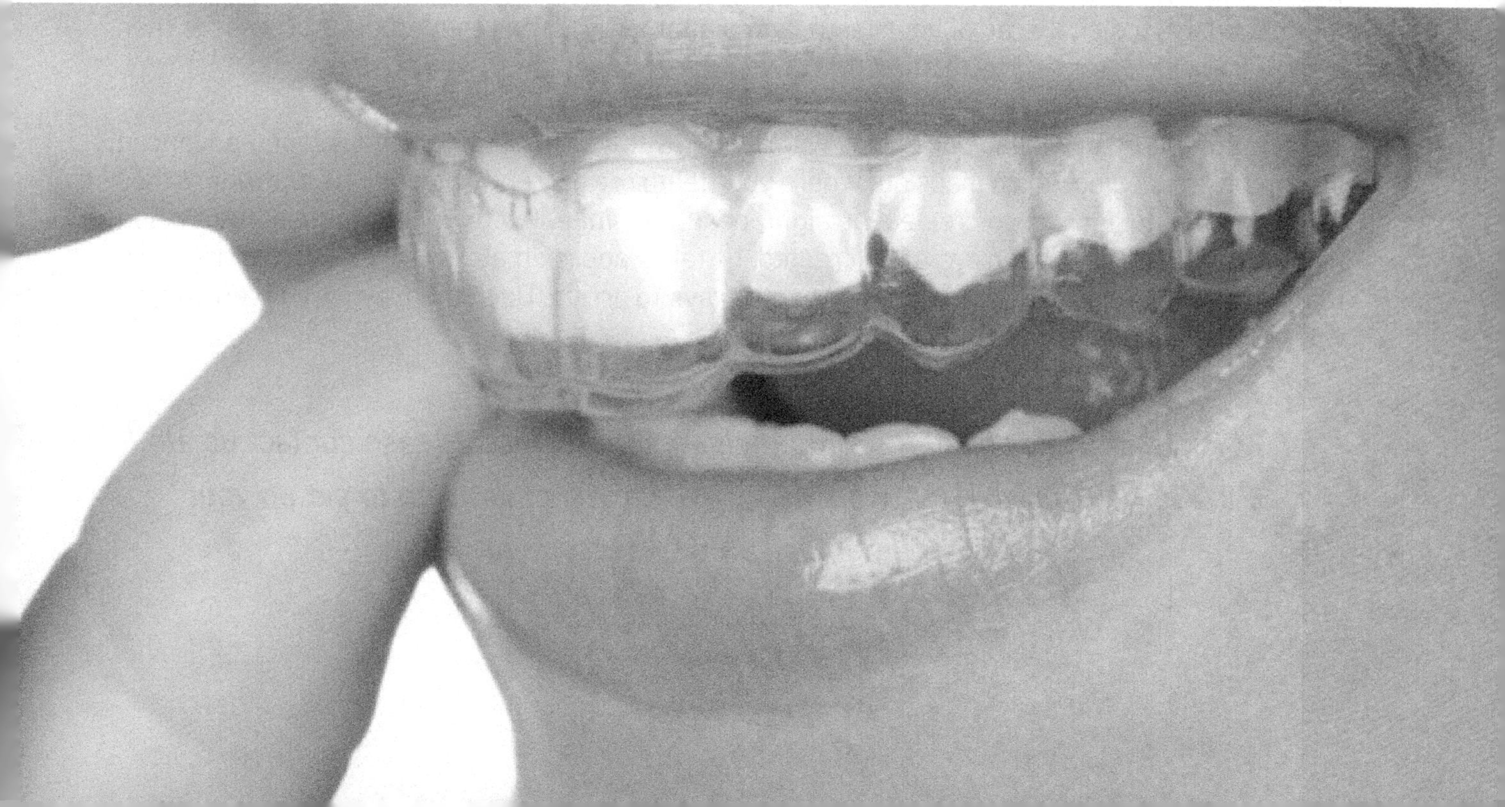

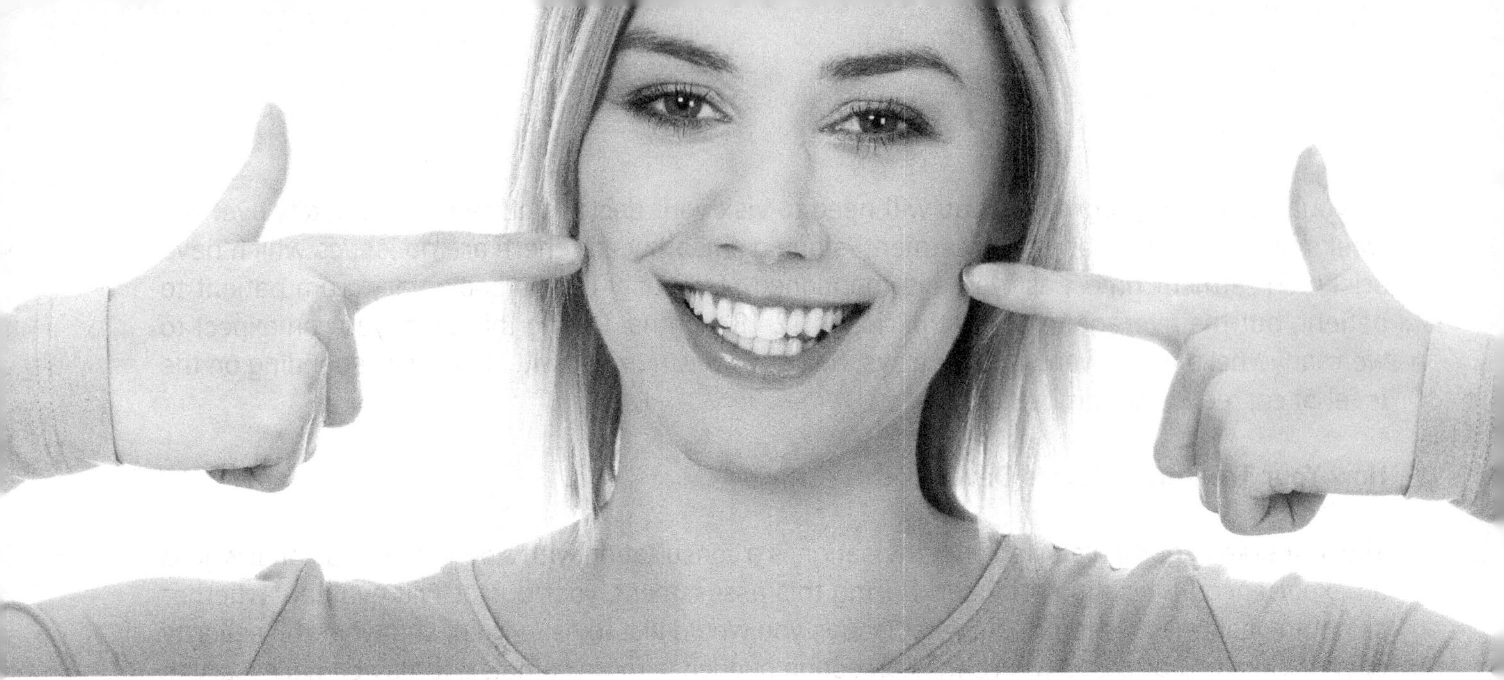

Once your doctor has determined that you are a good candidate for Invisalign, a series of steps will be taken to build records for your treatment. These steps include taking photographs of your teeth and face, a digital scan of your teeth, and digital x-rays. The result of each process is then sent to Invisalign to await the completion of your treatment plan by your doctor.

Your treatment plan, which your doctor will review with you in detail, includes using advanced 3D computer imaging which maps out where your teeth are currently positioned, and where they will be moved to in order to create a straight, beautiful smile. We then set the plan into motion by approving your aligner trays to be created. It takes approximately 4-5 weeks from the time that your initial impressions are made for your trays to arrive. Once the trays are received, you will be ready to begin your treatment.

TS Orthodontics is one of NC's top Invisalign providers. Please contact us at 828-254-4602 or visit our website at www.mytsosmile.com to set up your complimentary Smile Assessment.

How Your Aligners are Created

When Align Technology receives your x-rays, photos and treatment plan details, the process of creating your Invisalign aligner trays can begin.

To start the process, technicians generate a 3D model of a patient's mouth. This model is used to create a series of rendered simulations, which helps them mold your series of trays into the exact patterns and dimensions necessary to move your teeth into their final positions. These renderings provide a clear picture of how your smile will look at the end of your treatment. They also help determine how many trays will be needed throughout the course of your treatment. Your doctor will provide input to Align Technology in order to customize your treatment and to ensure a successful result.

Your aligners are then created, using a detailed and precise manufacturing process that is designed to provide you with the maximum amount of comfort while wearing them.

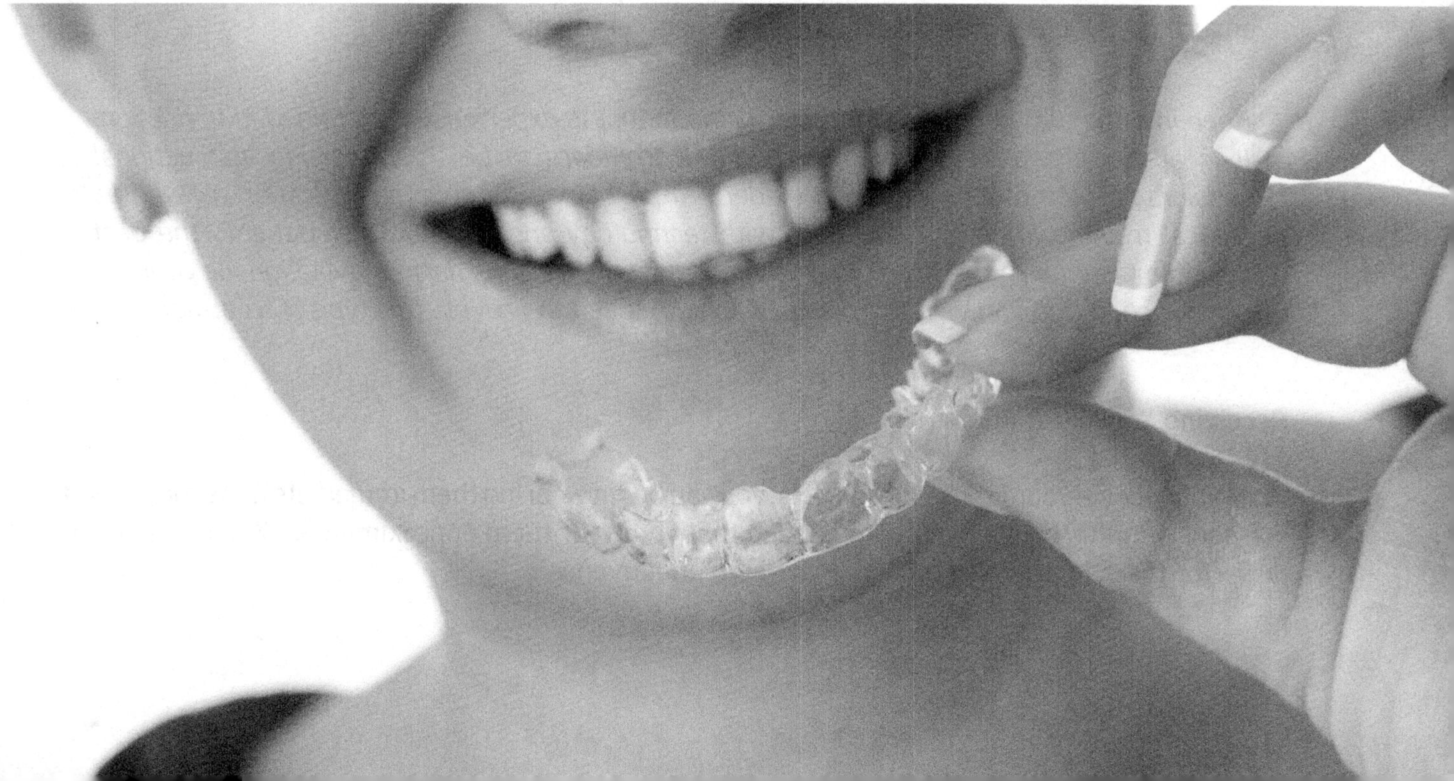

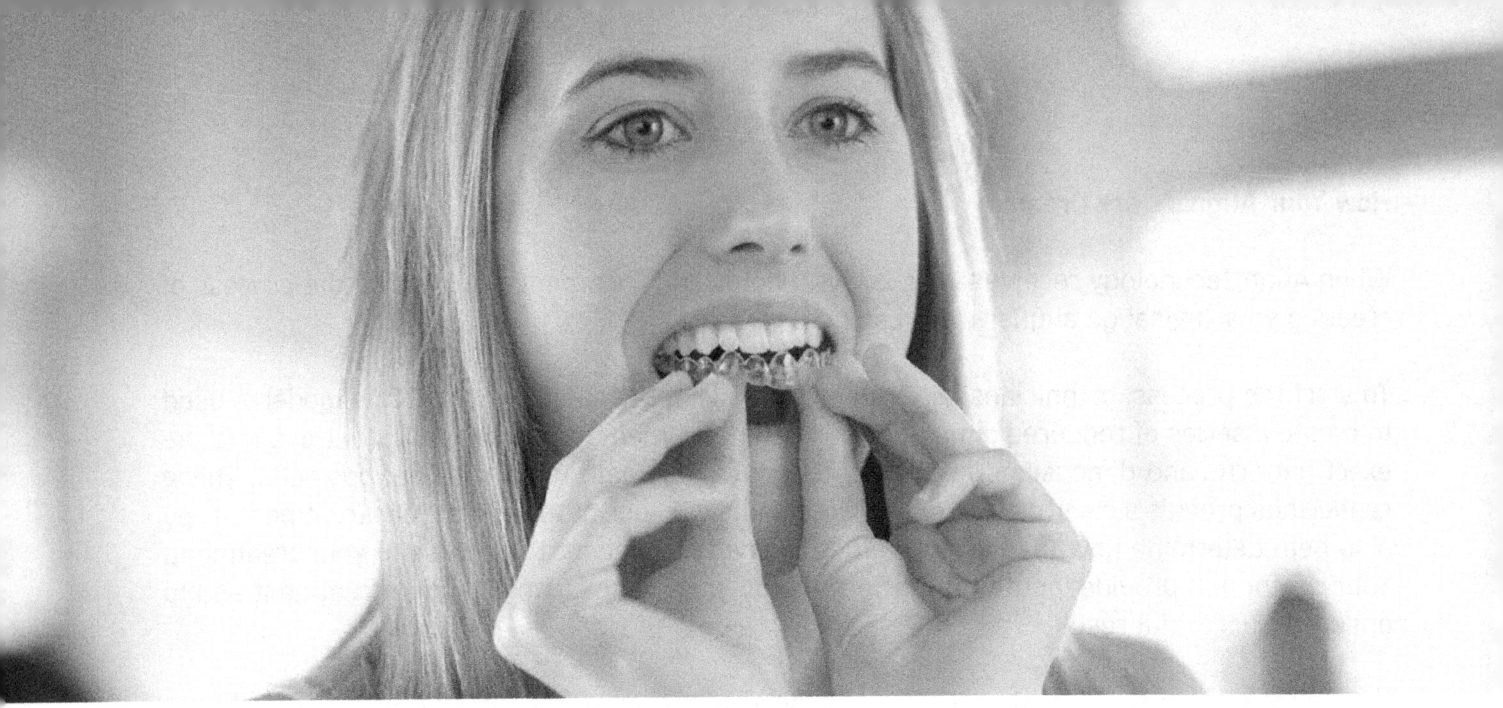

Because everyone's gum line is different, each aligner is individually trimmed for accuracy and comfort after creation. Before being provided to the patient, each tray is also checked for quality to ensure that you get the best results from your treatment.

Keep in mind that not every dentist or orthodontist is experienced or trained in Invisalign. It is a specialized treatment that requires providers to be trained using instructional sessions. It also requires those providers to participate in ongoing education as well as clinical training in order to keep up with technology and provide their patients the best possible treatment. Therefore, make sure that if you are considering Invisalign for yourself or your child that you visit a provider who is certified to provide this type of treatment.

Receiving Your First Aligners

Once you receive your first set of aligners, you can begin wearing them immediately. As mentioned previously in this book, it is recommended that you wear them approximately 22 hours a day in order for them to provide you with maximum effectiveness.

Approximately every two weeks, you will move on to a different set of aligners, which will move your teeth an additional 0.25mm from the previous tray. This process will continue until your teeth are in their ideal, straight positions.

Living with Clear Aligners

Besides aesthetic factors, one thing that patients find appealing about Invisalign versus traditional braces is that care and upkeep is easier to comply with. And while yes, your Invisalign aligners are unnoticeable to others and do not interrupt many facets of your daily life – there are still things that you must be mindful of in order for your treatment to be successful.

One of the most important things to be mindful of is that the better the patient compliance is, the better your results will be.

As part of your treatment, your doctor will go over what is expected of you as a patient in order to ensure your treatment is successful. There are also some general "dos-and-don'ts" that all patients who are undergoing treatment with Invisalign should follow as best practice. Some of those include:

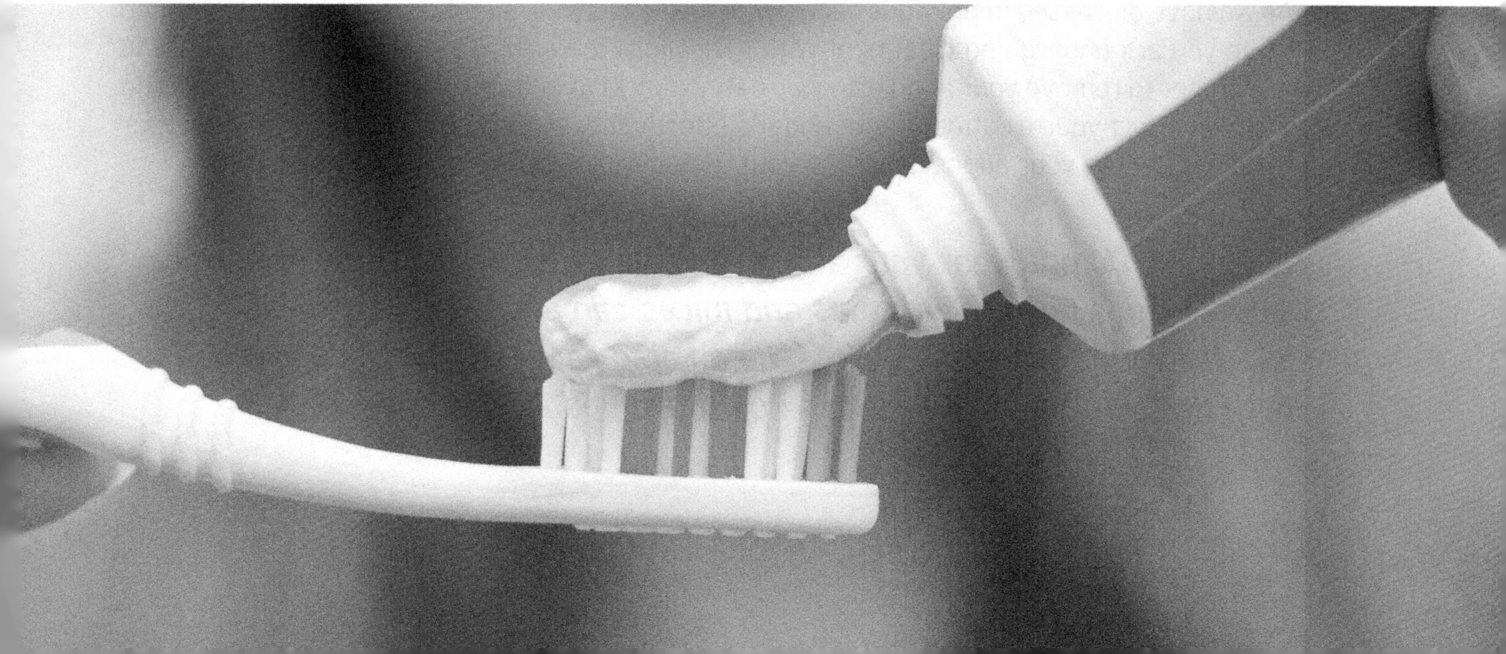

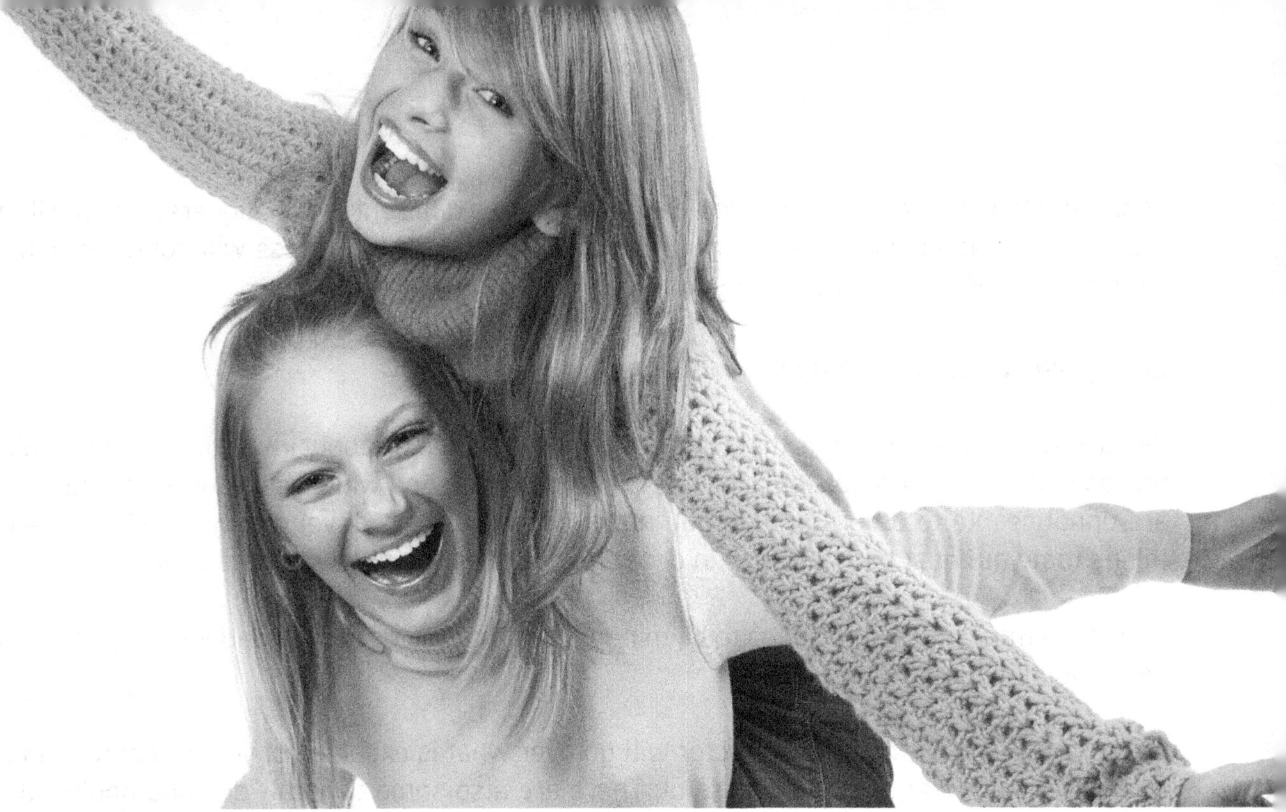

1. **DO remove your aligners when you eat**
   As we have discussed in previous sections of this book, your diet does not have to be limited while you are undergoing treatment with Invisalign However, it is very important that you remember to remove your aligners when eating any kind of food as it can damage them, and that will affect your treatment time and it's effectiveness. Also be sure to brush after your meal and secure your aligners back in your mouth quickly when you are done eating.

Reminder: Do not wear your aligners while drinking anything except water. Things like coffee, colas and juices can easily stain and/or discolor your aligners - quickly! It can also cause staining and even tooth decay to have these types liquid trapped in your trays.

2. **DO smile!**
   Even when wearing Invisalign, some people will still subconsciously hide their smile or cover their mouth when they speak to avoid having people notice their teeth. With Invisalign, you can smile with confidence! Most people will not even realize or notice that you are wearing braces!

3. **DO brush and floss your teeth frequently**
   When you are undergoing treatment with Invisalign, it is more important than ever to make sure that you keep up with your brushing and flossing routines - or that you improve them if this was not something you are already diligent about. You should aim to brush at least three times a day for best results, and floss one time a day. When you remove your aligners, be sure to clean them as well - a soft bristle brush is best. You may also safely soak them in denture cleaner.

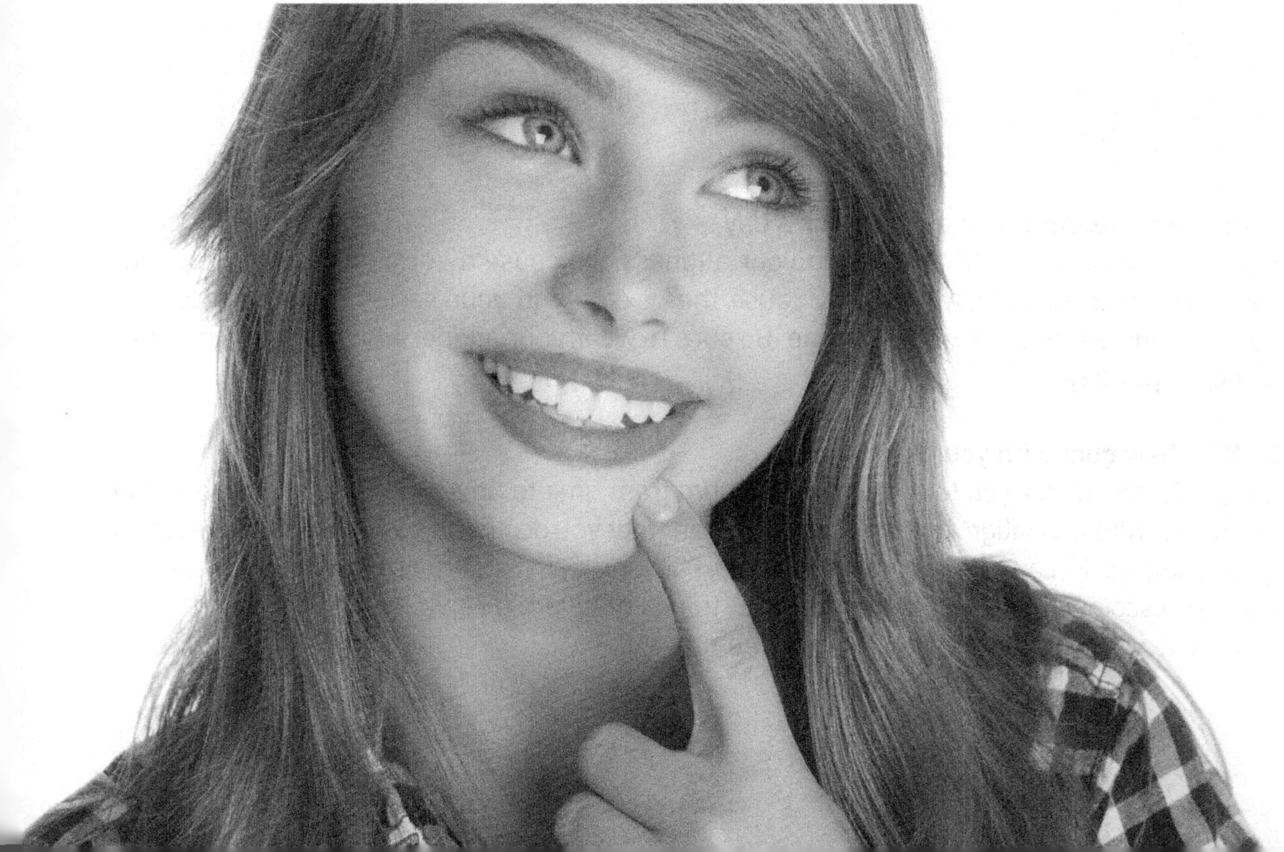

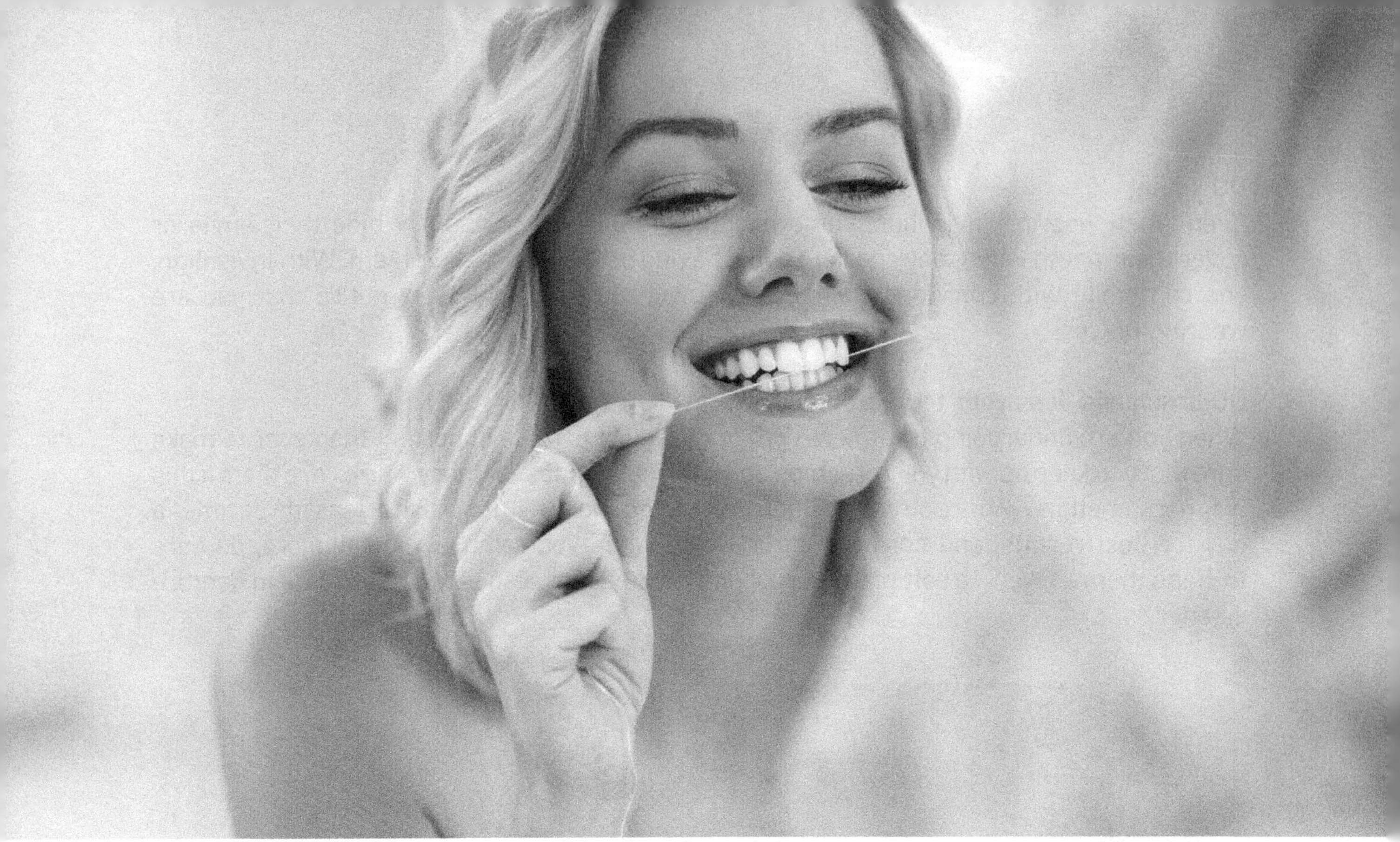

4. **DON'T skip wearing your aligners for a day**
   Skipping a day or a night of wearing your aligners can cause a serious disruption in your treatment schedule. It may not only cause the next tray in your series to not fit properly, but it can increase your treatment time. Be sure to wear your aligners for the recommended 22 hours per day.

5. **DON'T chew gum with your aligners in**
   It is perfectly fine for you to enjoy chewing gum from time to time while you are undergoing treatment with Invisalign, but it is very important that you do not do so while you are wearing your aligners. Because it is sticky by nature, chewing gum can adhere to your aligners and not just discolor them, but damage them to the point where a replacement is needed. This will cause you to suffer a delay in your treatment time.

Your Treatment Timeline

For both teens and adults, the treatment time for straightening teeth using Invisalign takes an average of 12-18 months, depending on the severity of the case. Much like the aligners themselves are custom made, your treatment plan will be also - the doctor will work closely with you to determine a timeline using a method that best fulfills your individual needs.

Keep in mind that because all patients are different, so is their treatment - and their treatment times. While it is not unusual for some people to complete their treatment in less than the projected time, it is not typical. The process of correction is not one that can be rushed and it is advised that you always follow the guidelines provided to you by your doctor.

It won't be long before you start seeing results once your treatment begins - in fact, one of Invisalign's features that patients enjoy the most is the ability to see your smile correction in real time. You will start seeing changes after a couple of months if not sooner. When treatment is complete, there is no "big reveal" moment. You don't have to wonder what your smile will ultimately look like because you are able to see that every step of the way. This is something that is not possible with traditional braces, giving Invisalign a clear advantage in being able to see progress in a shorter amount of time.

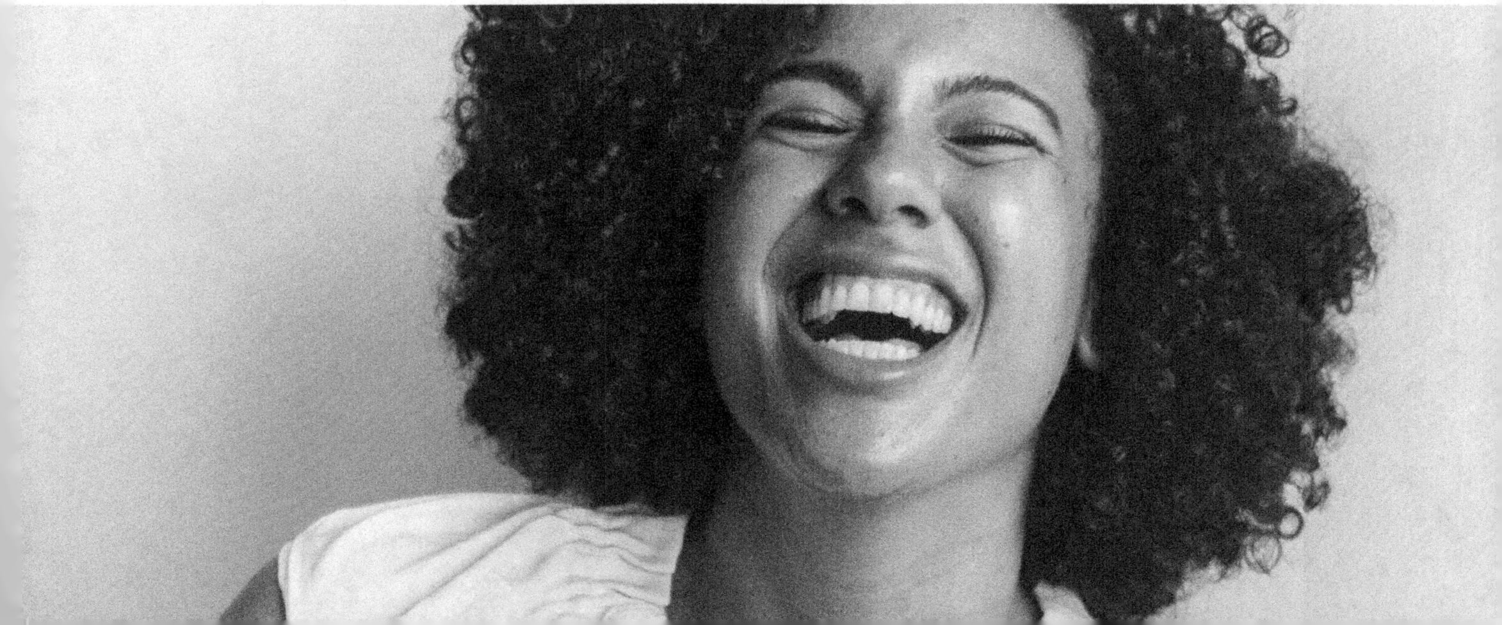

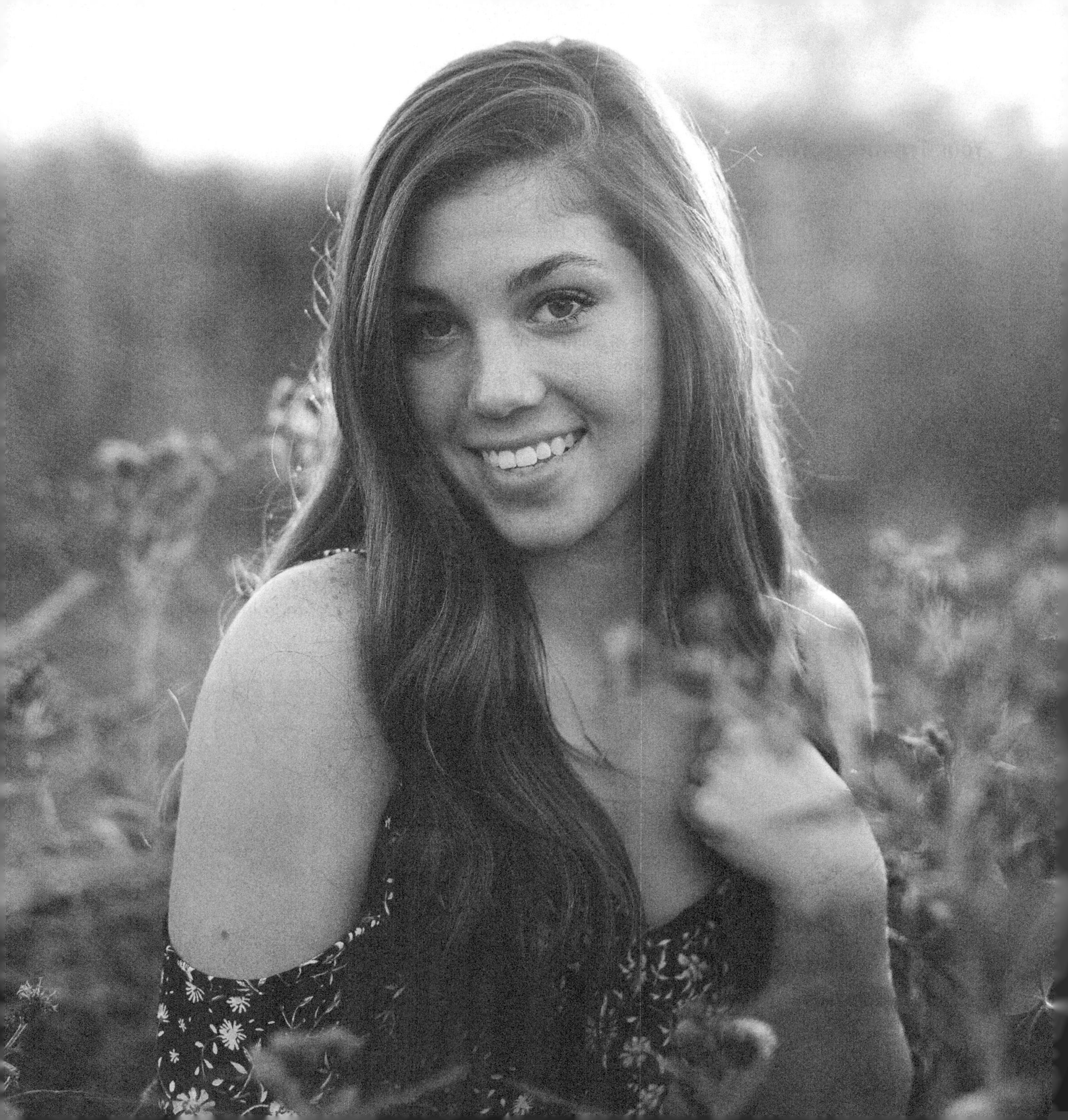

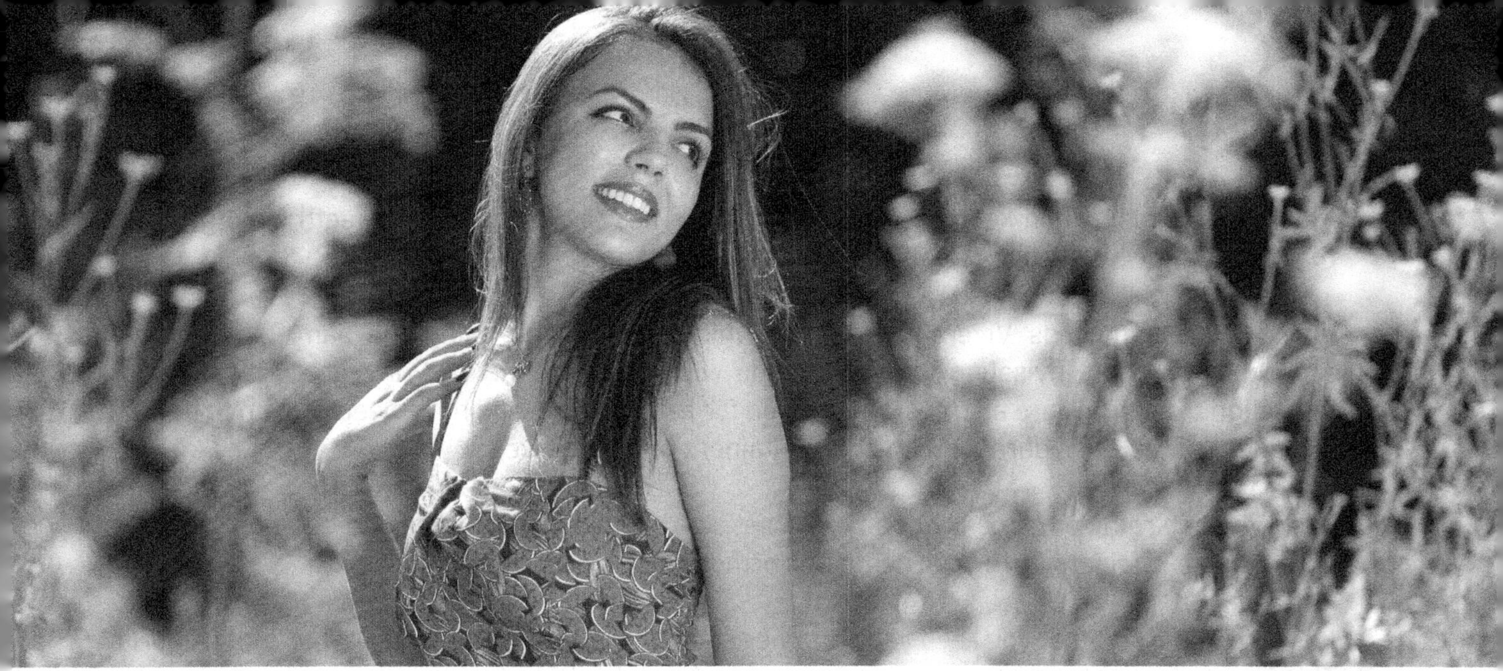

Post Treatment Care

Once you complete your Invisalign treatment, you will have a beautiful, straight smile that you will want to show off to everyone. In order to keep it looking it's best, it is important to know that proper steps must be taken in order to keep it looking it's best for a lifetime.

Once your treatment is complete, your doctor may recommend that you wear retainers for a period of time (This is a requirement for any type of braces, including traditional metal ones). This is because, unfortunately, teeth can shift back towards their pre-treatment positions when that extra support is not provided.

After spending a lot of time and money on their smile, many patients see it as an investment. Retainer wear is protection for that investment.

It cannot be emphasized enough that it is very important for you to wear your retainer as directed by your doctor when you complete your treatment. This is critical for keeping the tension on your teeth that will hold them in place.

Retainers do more than keep your teeth straight. They also protect your teeth from grinding them at night, which causes wear and tear and even damage to your teeth.

Invisalign recommends Vivera® retainers, which are created using the same state-of-the-art technology that Invisalign trays are made with. They are virtually invisible just like your Invisalign trays. They are also custom-created for each patient, and have been proven to be 30% stronger and twice as durable than other retainers on the market.

Each Vivera® retainer comes with an extra set as a replacement in case one gets lost. You can obtain these retainers from your dentist or orthodontist's office.

It is also important that you keep your retainer clean to prevent the build up of harmful bacteria. This is very important to do in order to keep your teeth healthy.

Do not use toothpaste to clean your retainers. Because of it's abrasive nature, it can damage your retainer and dull it's shine, which can lead to stained teeth and excessive germ build up.

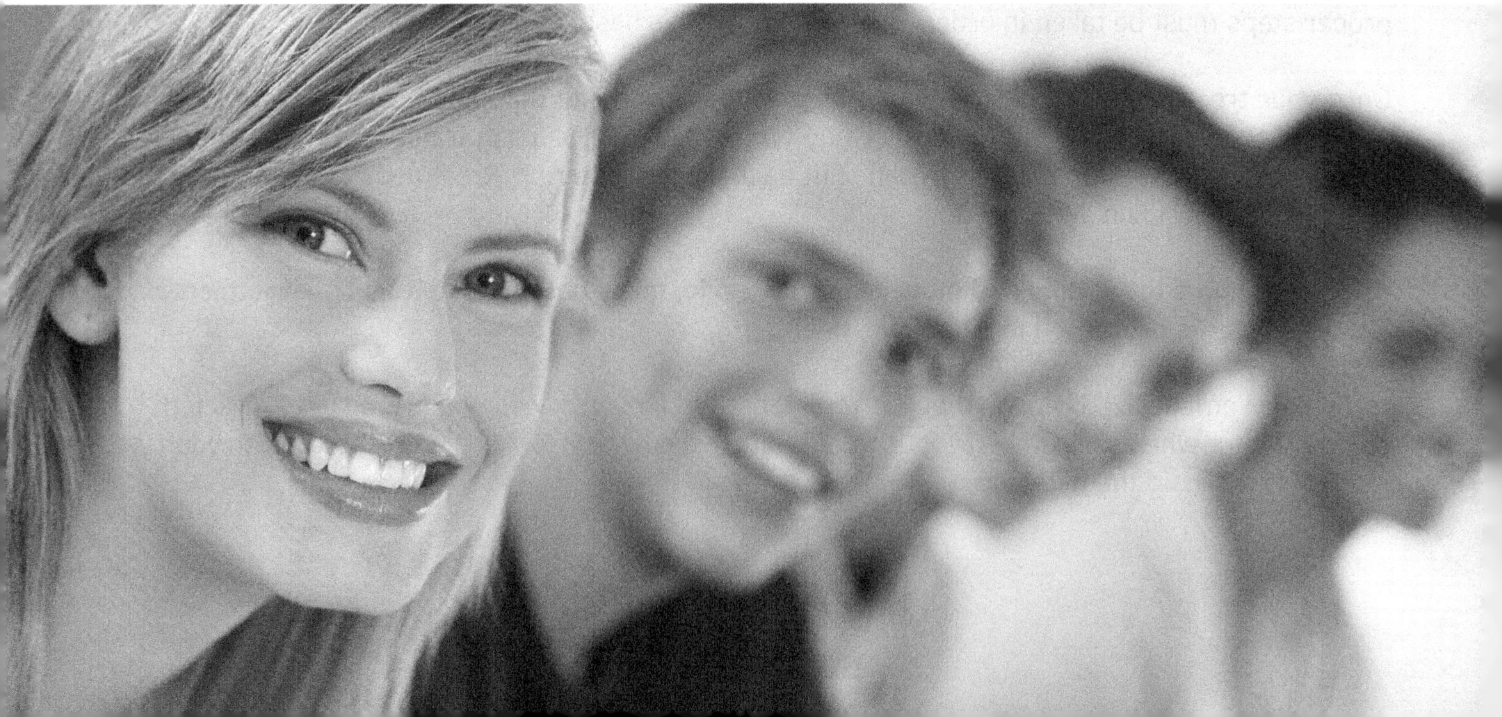

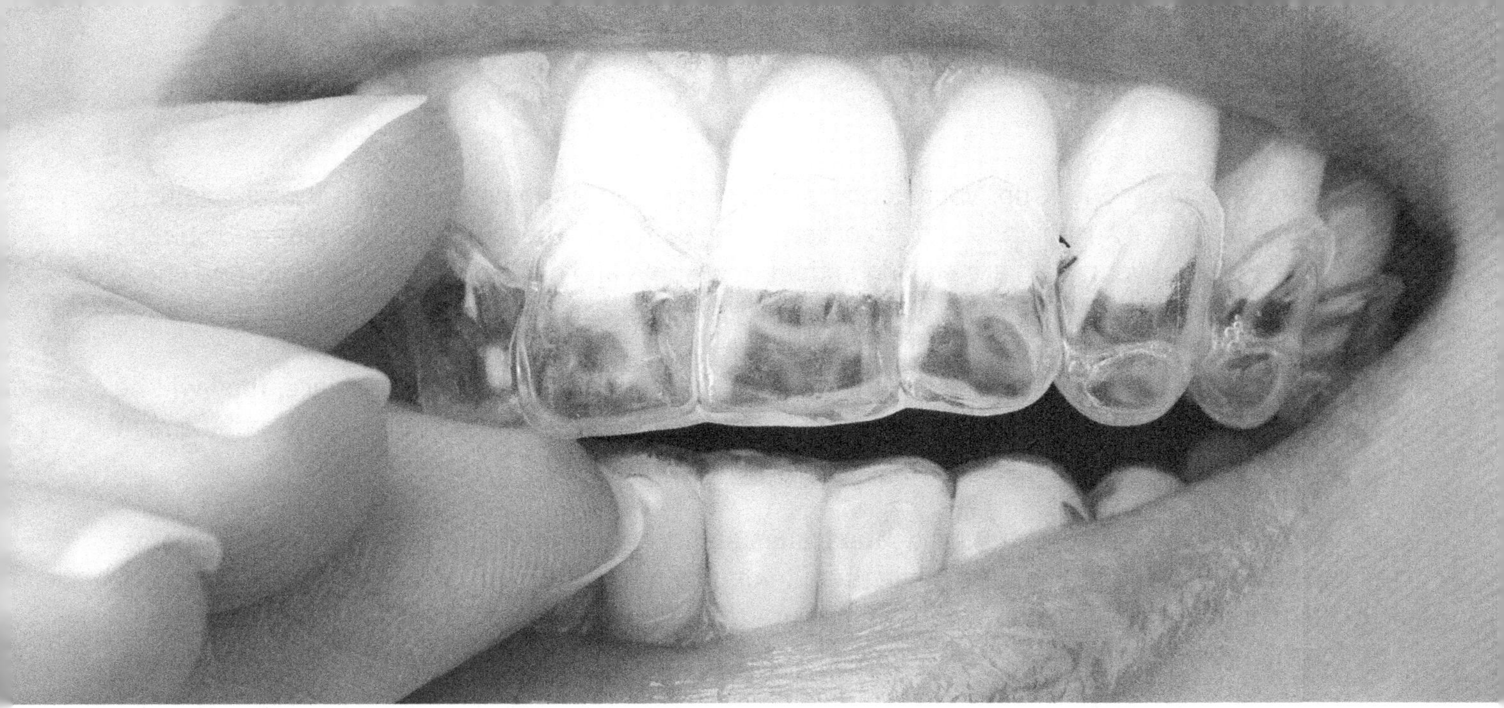

There are several ways to safely clean your retainers which will keep them in good shape and working properly. One is to clean it using warm soapy water, scrubbing it gently with a toothbrush. This should be done each day for maximum effectiveness. Be sure to rinse the retainer after your cleaning is complete.

Another option is to purchase tablets which are specially formulated to clean retainers. Using them is simple and similar to the way that dentures are cleaned - simply drop a tablet into a cup of water each day and place your retainer in the water. The solution will work to break down any bacteria that is on the retainer. The recommended time to keep your retainer submerged is ten to twenty minutes a day. The tablet solution is not abrasive or damaging to the retainers composition, so it may be left submerged for longer than that; however a ten to twenty minute cleaning is all that is necessary to get the retainer ready to put in your mouth.

After you complete your Invisalign treatment, don't forget to schedule regular dental checkups. These are important for everyone, but they are especially important for a former Invisalign patient.

During a routine check up, your dental professional can examine your overall oral health to make sure that everything is in good order post treatment. They will also examine your bite to make sure that your teeth are staying in their new spots and not crowding or shifting, and check to see your bite's stability.

If your dentist notes that some of your teeth are shifting and moving out of place, they will be able evaluate and adjust your retainer wear if it is needed, as well as provide a replacement should your current one be damaged or otherwise ineffective.

Invisalign can help correct your dental issues and provide you with the smile of your dreams, but maintaining that beautiful smile is a lifelong commitment. With just a few good post care habits that are easy to follow, you can be sure to keep your new smile looking it's absolute best for many years to come.

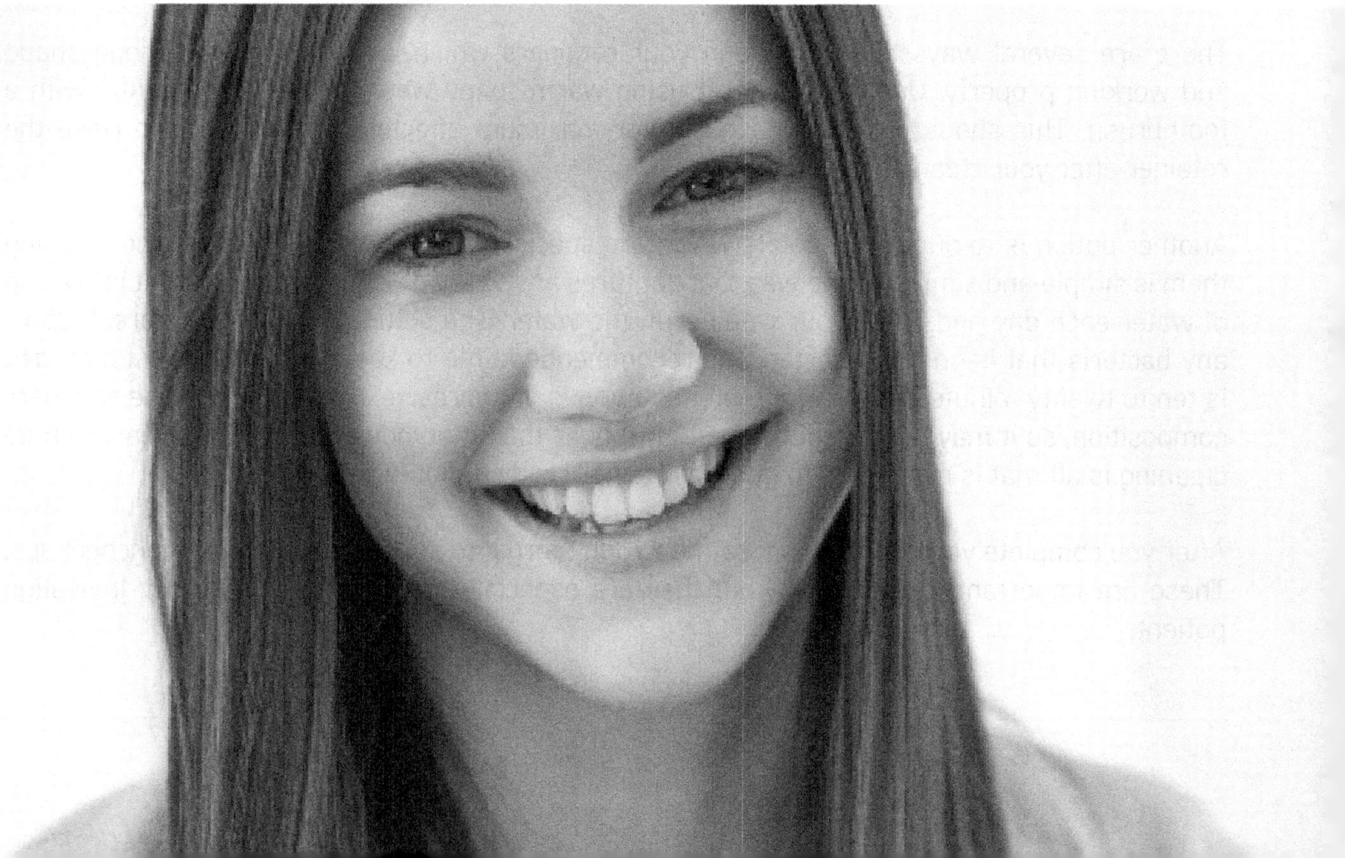

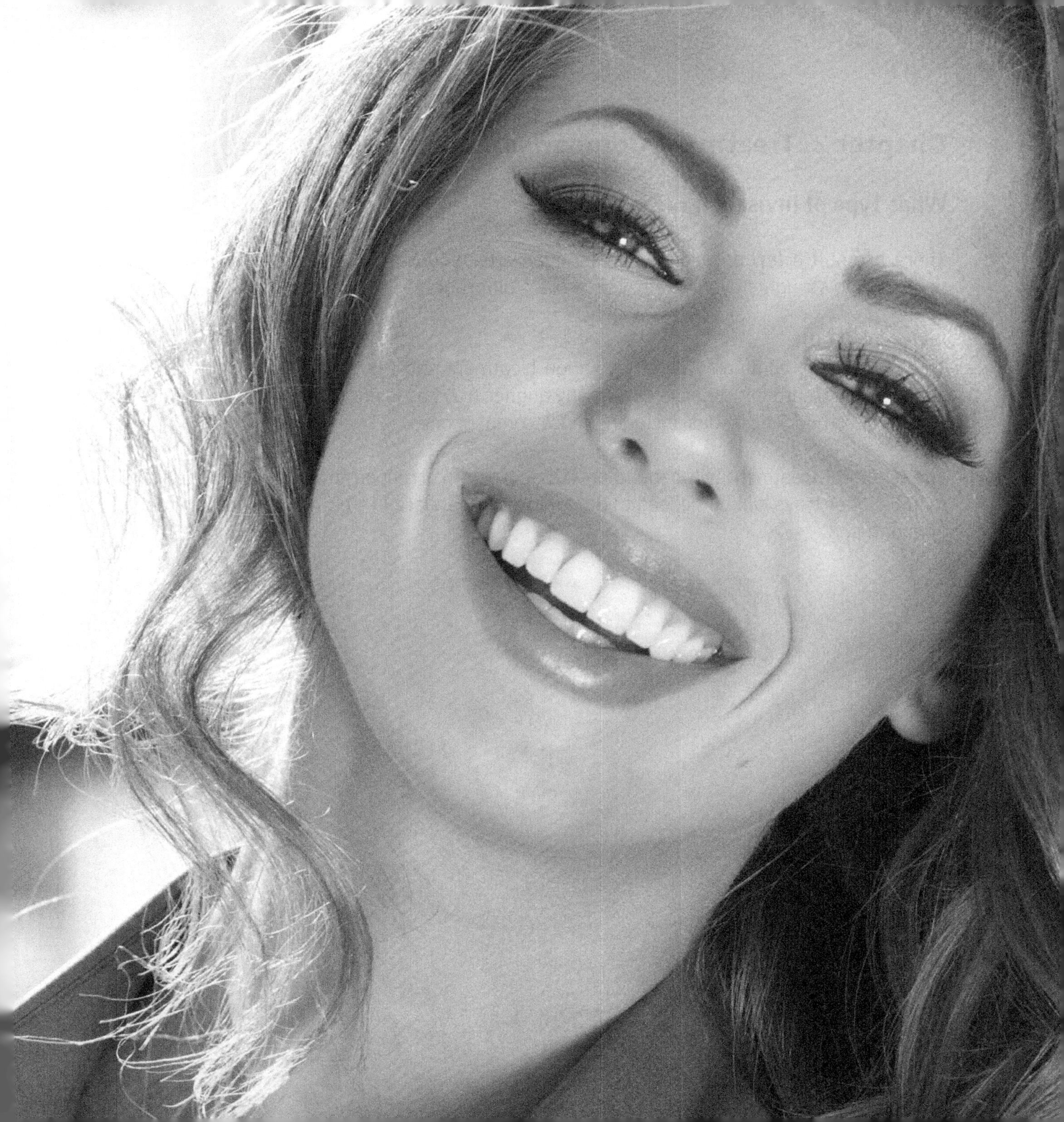

Chapter 3: Treatment Comparisons

What Type of Invisalign is Right for Me?

There are still a few decisions to make even after you have decided that you want to have Invisalign to straighten your teeth. There are 4 different types to choose from:

Invisalign (Full)
This is the most common type of Invisalign treatment and the one that a majority of patients choose. This treatment consiste of as many aligner trays as is necessary in order to fully treat a variety of orthodontic issues, including more complex ones.

The length of treatment will depend on the degree of correction that must be done - and how many aligner trays will be needed to do it. Most patients are in treatment for an average of 12-18 months.

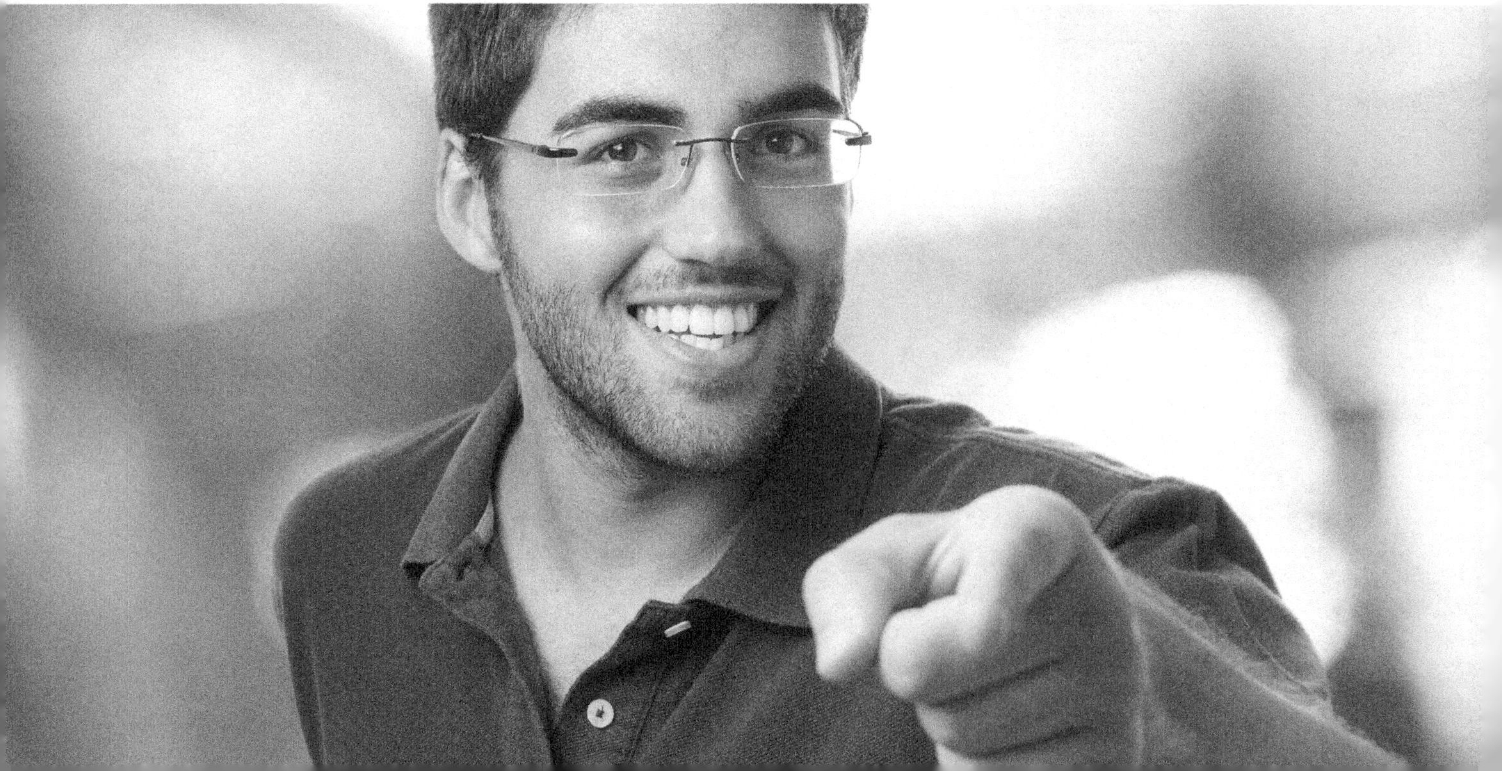

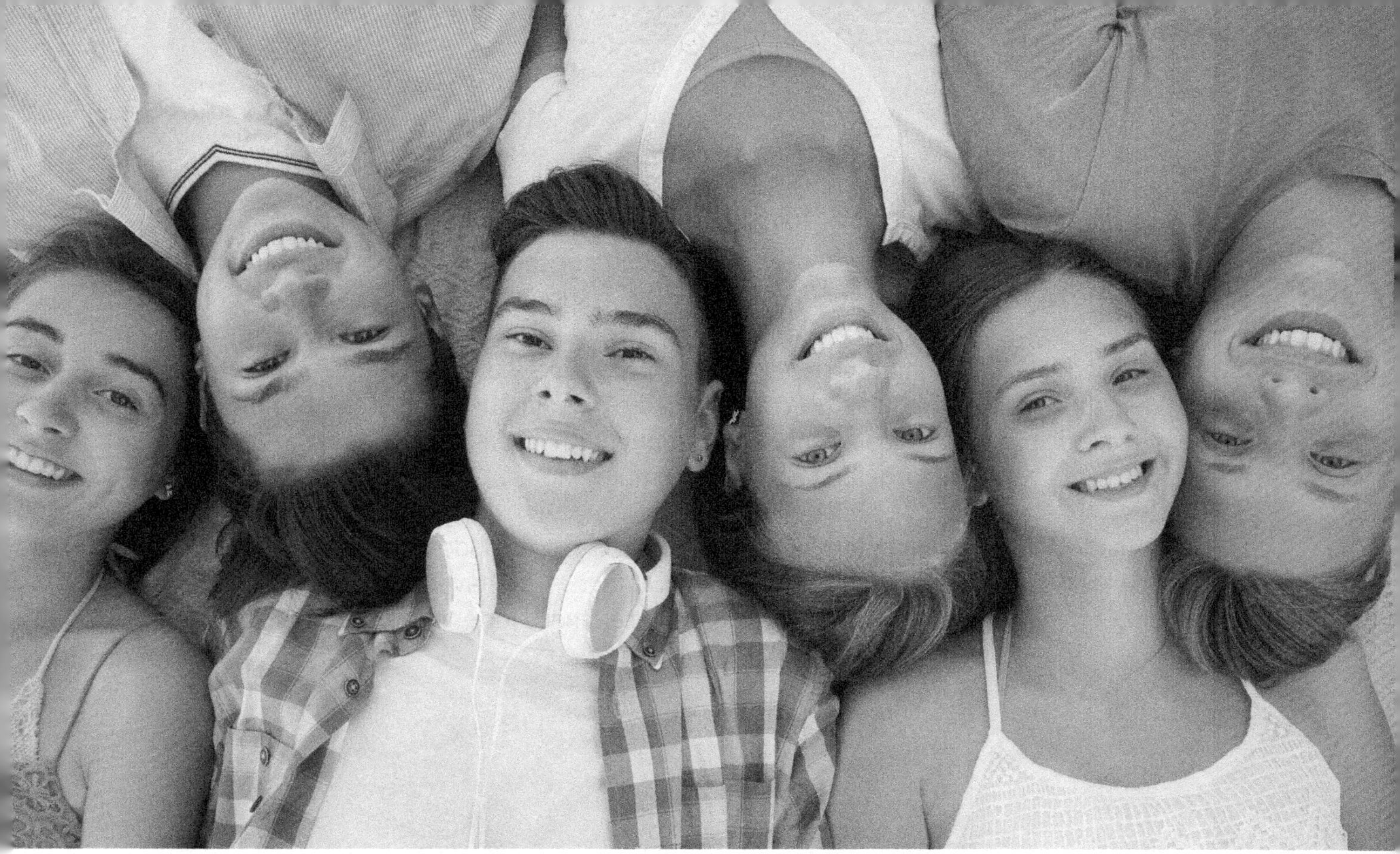

Invisalign Lite

This treatment is designed for simple cases where the alignment problem is minor and there are no other serious dental issues present, such as an overbite or crowding.

Invisalign Lite uses a fixed number of clear aligners to make these simple corrections and treatment time is usually only a couple of months.

Ideal for those who need the positioning of their teeth adjusted and straightened before they can have cosmetic work such as crowns or veneers, Invisalign Lite provides an easy and quick solution for patients who require a small amount of correction and wish to have it done in a minimal time period.

Invisalign i7

The newest offering from Align Technologies, Invisalign i7 is the quickest of the Invisalign treatment options. This solution can be used for adults or teens, and is for people who require minor tooth correction and have slight overcrowding issues.

Invisalign i7 aligners straighten your teeth by applying pressure on specific teeth at different times. The aligners are manufactured individually manufactured just as regular Invisalign aligners are, but they are focused only on straightening specific teeth. They are worn in two week increments, until the targeted teeth have completed the straightening process.

This treatment is ideal for people who have had previous orthodontic treatment or braces in the past so they do not need major correction work done – but have found that their teeth have shifted either due to age or due to not having worn retainers for enough time after treatment.

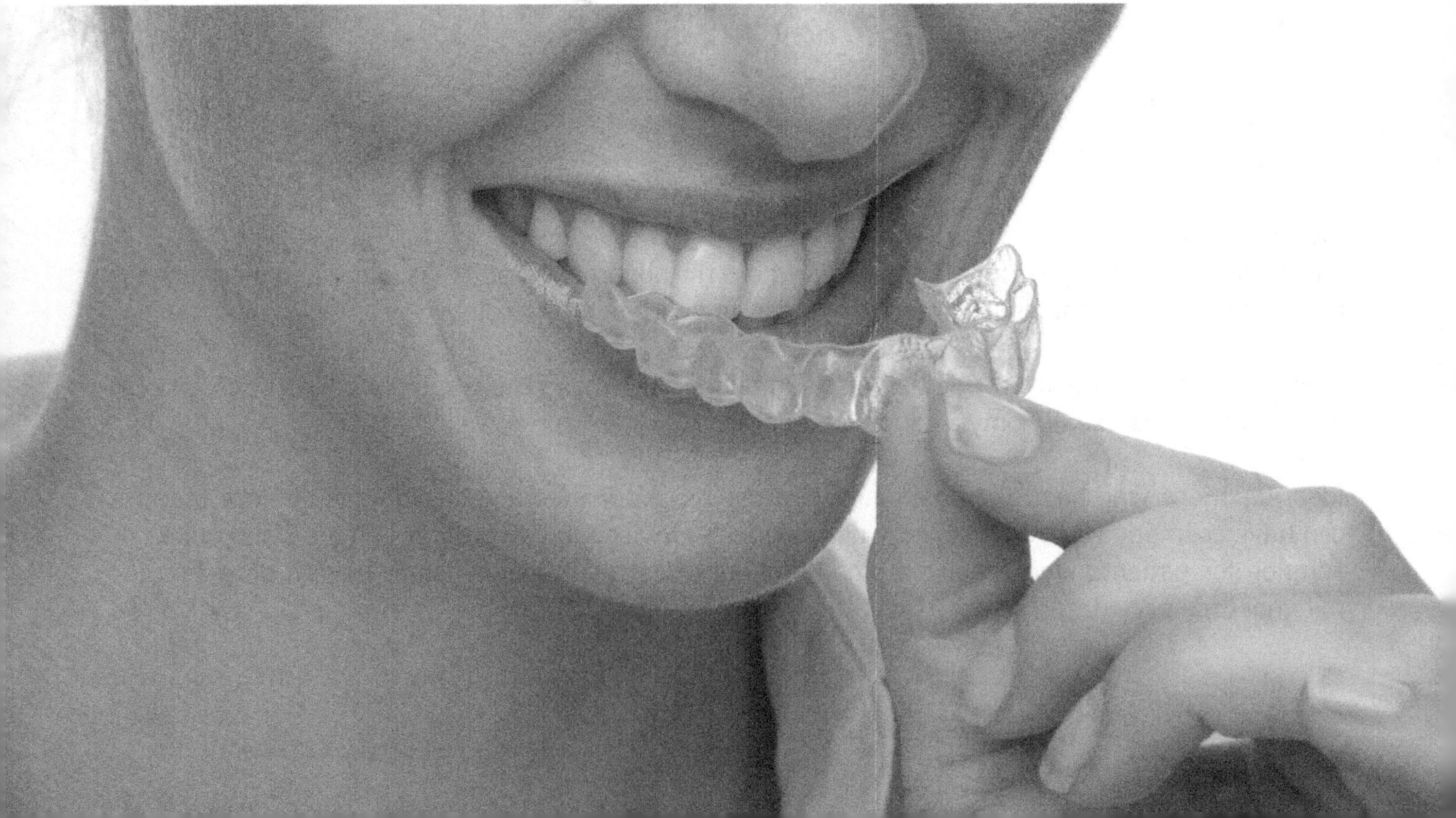

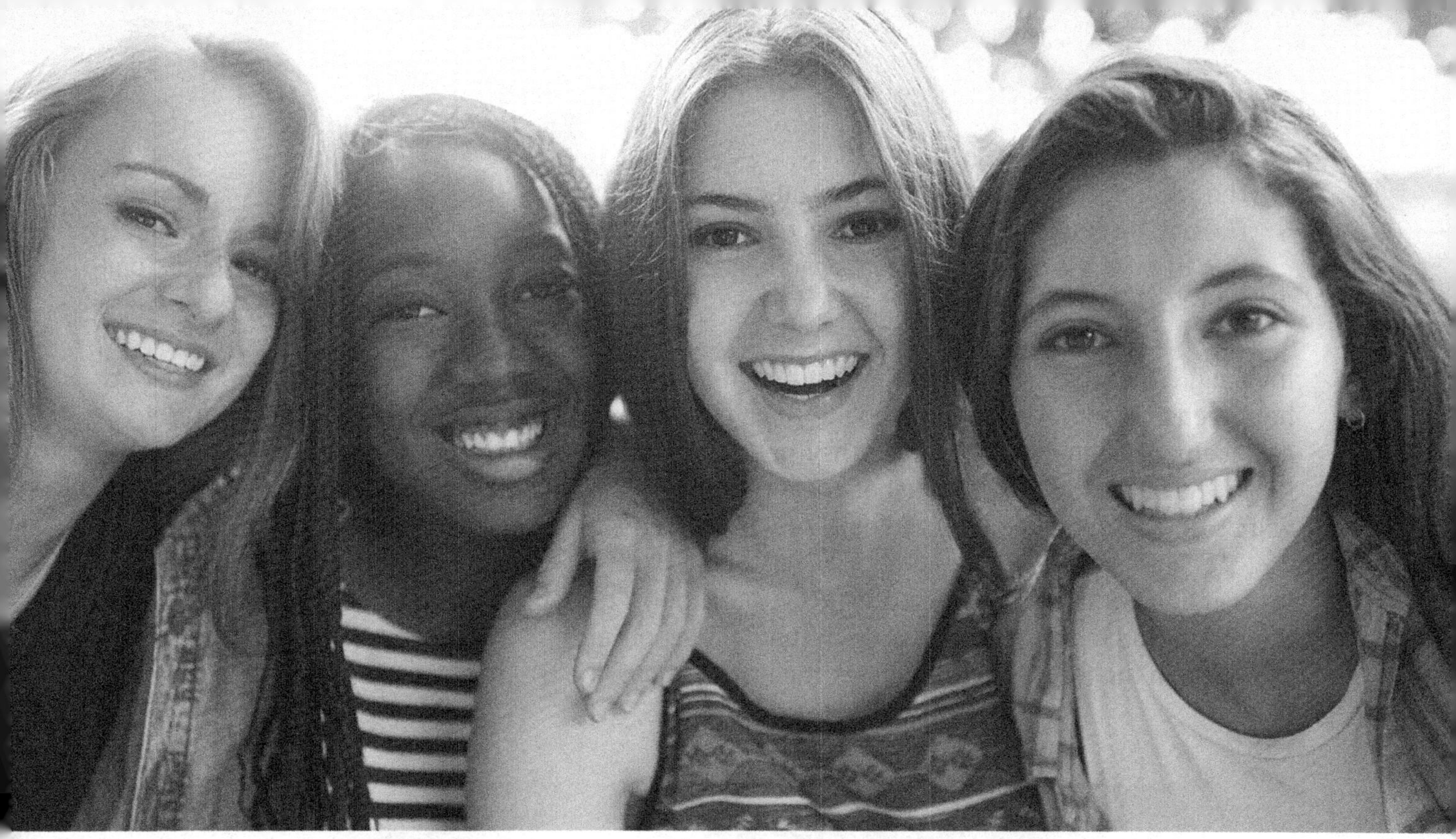

Invisalign Teen

This treatment is designed, as the name implies, especially for teens. Ages for this treatment can range from as young as eleven or twelve up, until age seventeen to eighteen, but it goes on a case by case basis as several factors must be present in order for a child to be a candidate for treatment.

The following factors must be present in order for a teen to be eligible:

- They must have lost all of their baby teeth
- All permanent molars and incisors must have erupted. The teen's second and third molars (known as wisdom teeth) do not have to be have erupted yet, as Invisalign trays can be created with room for those to come in over time.

- There cannot be any tooth decay or other damage present
- The patient must be able to comply with treatment stipulations, meaning that they must be able to wear the aligners every day and understand that they must remain in for 22 hours per day.

Invisalign Teen has some special features that the adult version does not have in order to help teens be compliant and complete their treatment successfully. This includes up to 6 free replacement aligner trays in case they get lost or damaged. This eliminates a parent's worry that if the child accidentally washes their aligners in shirt pocket or misplaces it at school, they will be able to obtain a quick and easy replacement so their treatment stays on track.

Invisalign Teen is also equipped with tooth eruption tabs that are designed to accommodate the rest of the teen's permanent teeth that will erupt later on in life. This prevents issues with crowding in the future and eliminates the need to have the treatment done again when they are older.

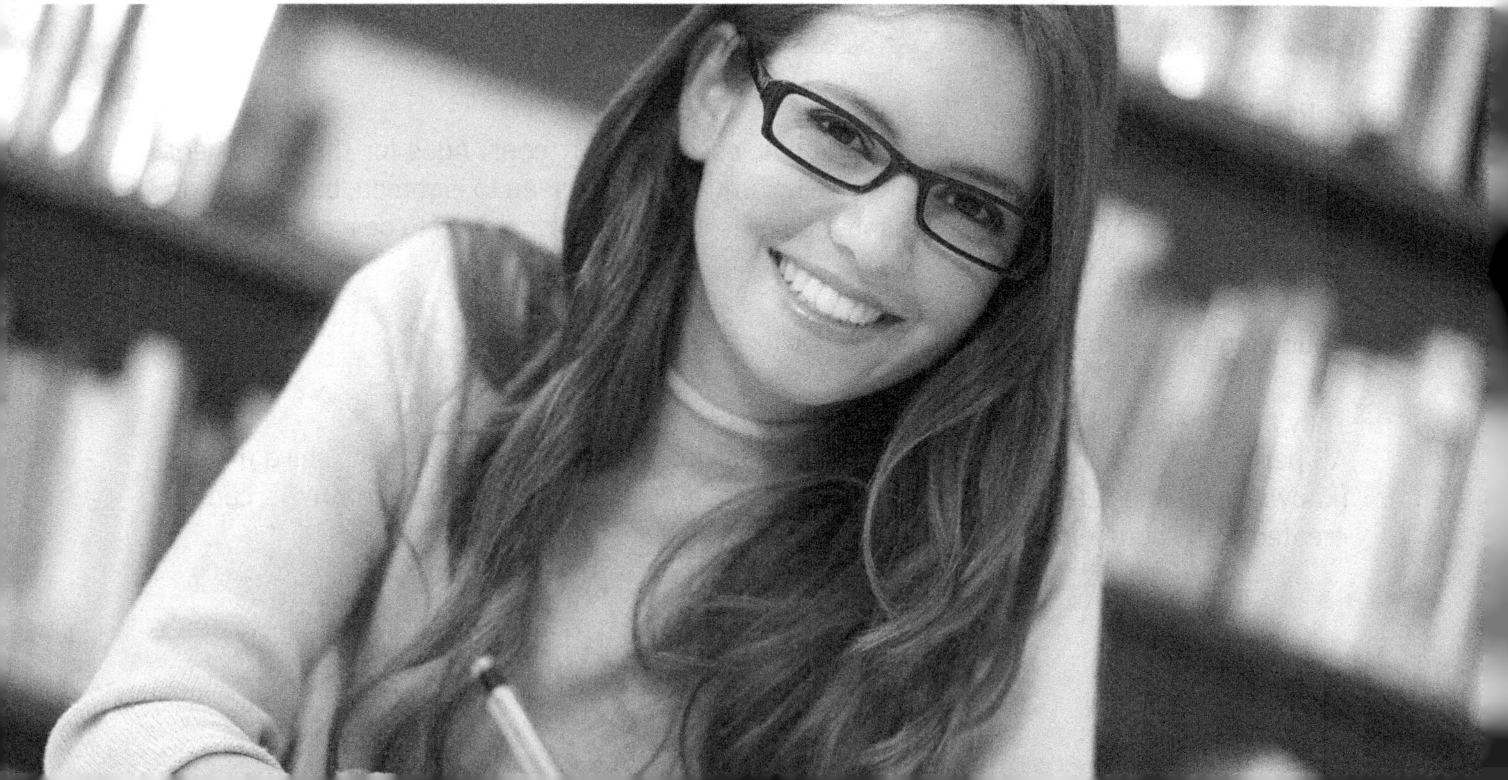

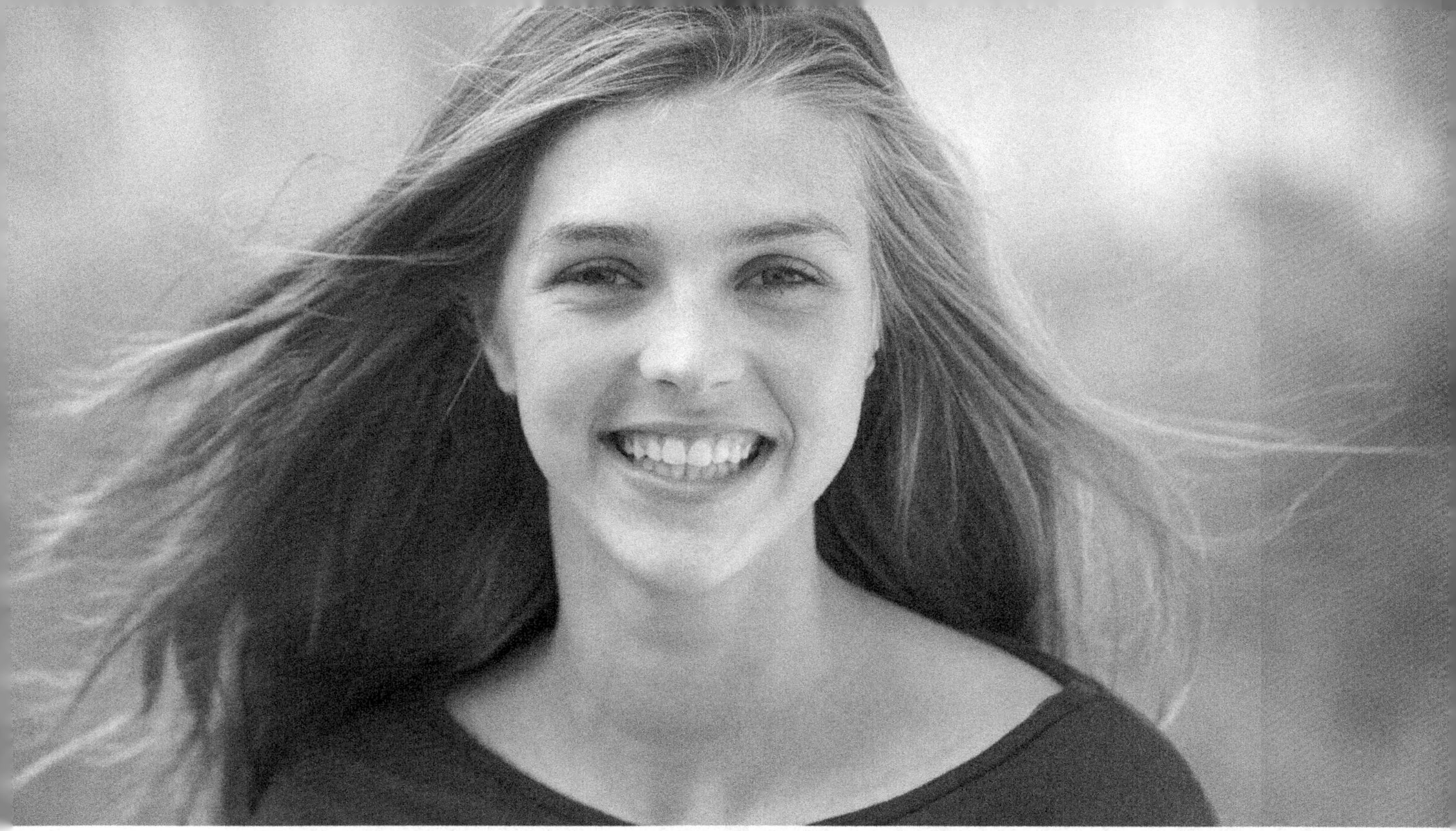

One of doctors' preferred features of Invisalign Teen is the blue compliance indicators that are embedded into the aligner trays. These sensors fade from blue to clear as the aligners are worn, and will help both the dentist and the teen's parent determine if the child is wearing the aligners for the proper amount of time each day.

Whether or not a teen is ready for treatment with Invisalign depends not just on physical factors but also on the level of maturity of the particular child. Most children beyond the ages of eleven to twelve are perfectly capable of handling the responsibilities that treatment entails. There are always cases where a child is absent minded and struggles with compliance, however, so it is important for them to be made aware of the importance of responsibility for their treatment.

For more information on Invisalign Teen, please see the section in this book titled "Treatment for Teens."

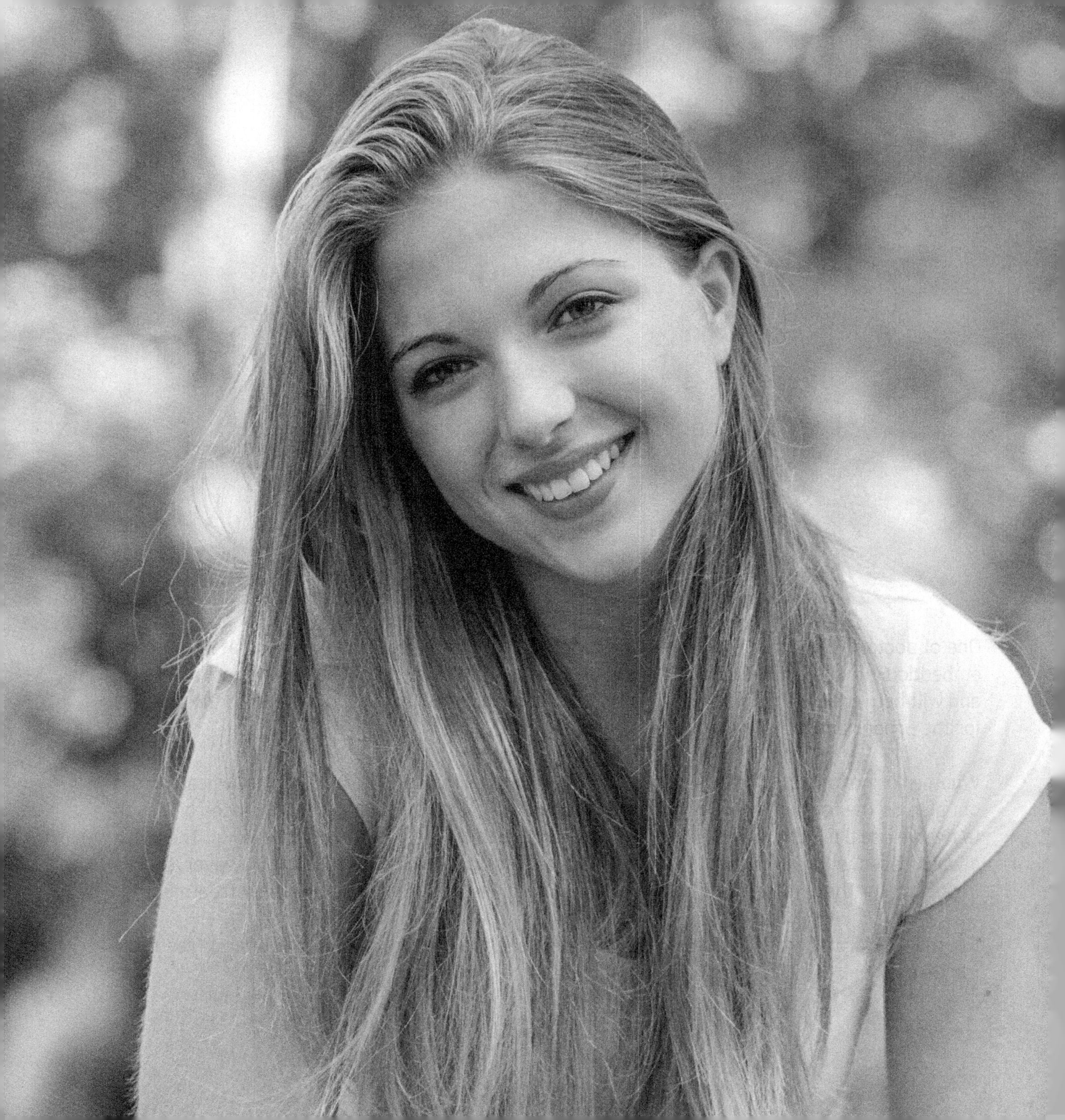

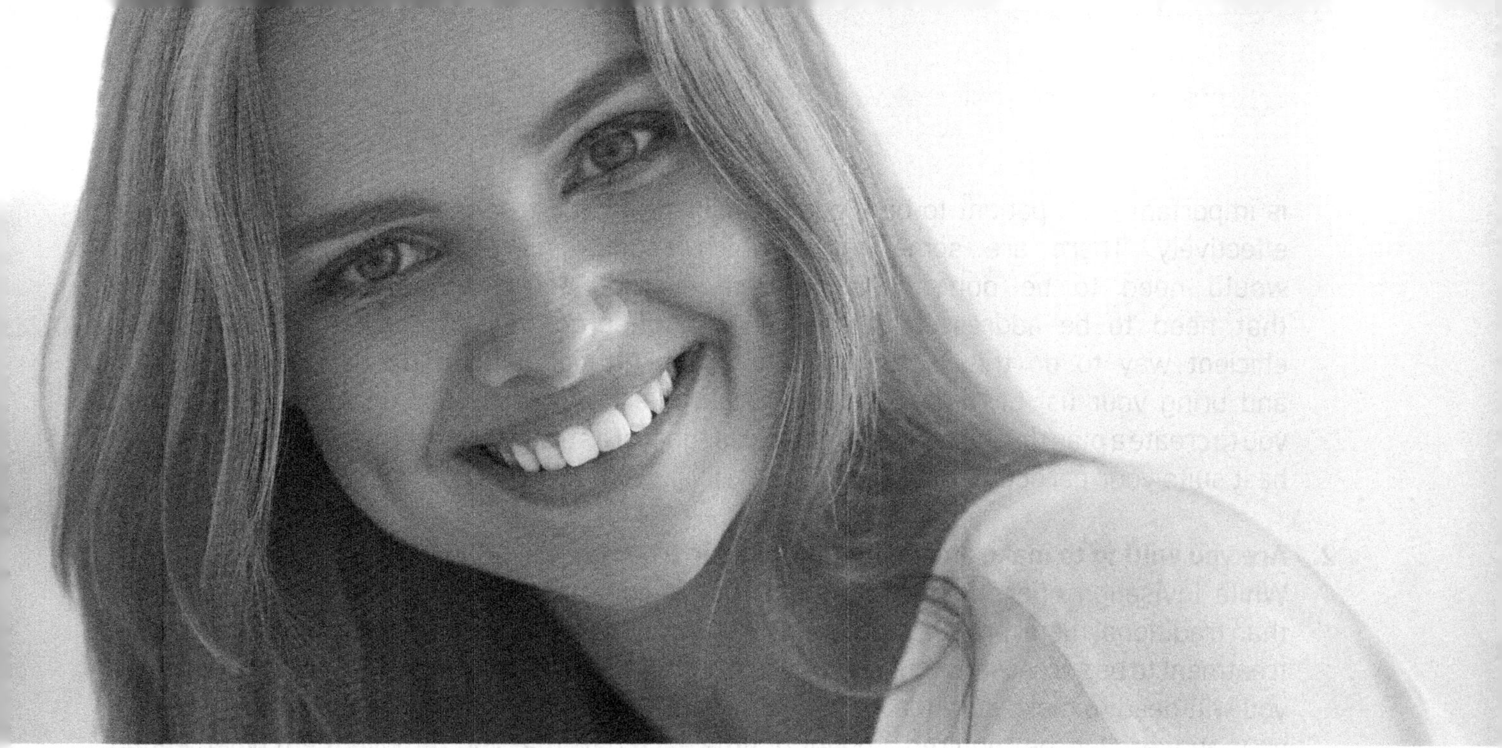

Questions to Ask Yourself About Invisalign

If you are considering braces for yourself or your child, this book provides you with a lot of information that will help you make a decision about your available options and what your "smile goals" are. While Invisalign is a great way to correct most issues with crooked teeth, it is not always the perfect solution for everyone. Some effort is needed from the patient as well to make the treatment a success.

Here are five basic questions that you should ask yourself in order to determine if Invisalign is best for you and the smile that you wish to achieve.

1. **What do you want to improve about your smile?**
   The first question you should ask yourself is what issues you feel you have with your smile, and what specific things you want to correct. Invisalign is, as we have discussed in previous chapters, a highly effective way to correct many issues with a less than perfect smile, but it

is important for a patient to be a good candidate for the treatment in order for it to work effectively. There are some cases which require more advanced correction that would need to be done in a different method (such as traditional braces) or that need to be addressed before you can undergo Invisalign treatment. The most efficient way to do this is to schedule a consultation with a dentist or orthodontist and bring your list of things that you would like to correct. Your doctor will work with you to create a plan that will help you get to your goal of a straight, beautiful smile in the way that best suits your particular situation.

2. **Are you willing to make a commitment to your treatment?**
   While Invisalign offers you a treatment that is comparatively less of a time investment than traditional metal braces, there are still things that you must comply with in order for your treatment to be successful. Your doctor will develop a specific treatment plan for you, however, you will need to make sure that you comply with the basics such as ensuring that you wear your aligners for the required amount of time each day, that you remove them when eating or drinking, and that you show up for your appointments to make sure your treatment is progressing. Like with any regiment that improves your health, Invisalign is a commitment, but it is one that most patients agree is well worth it.

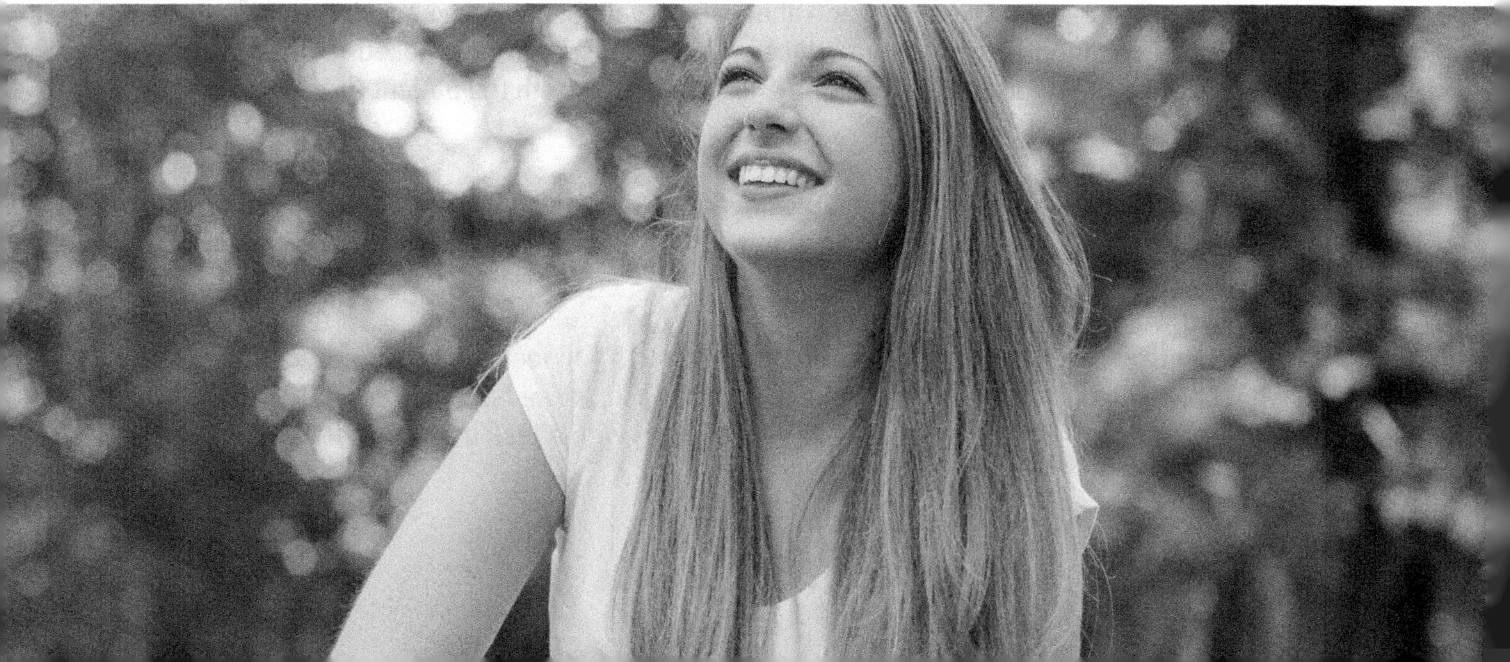

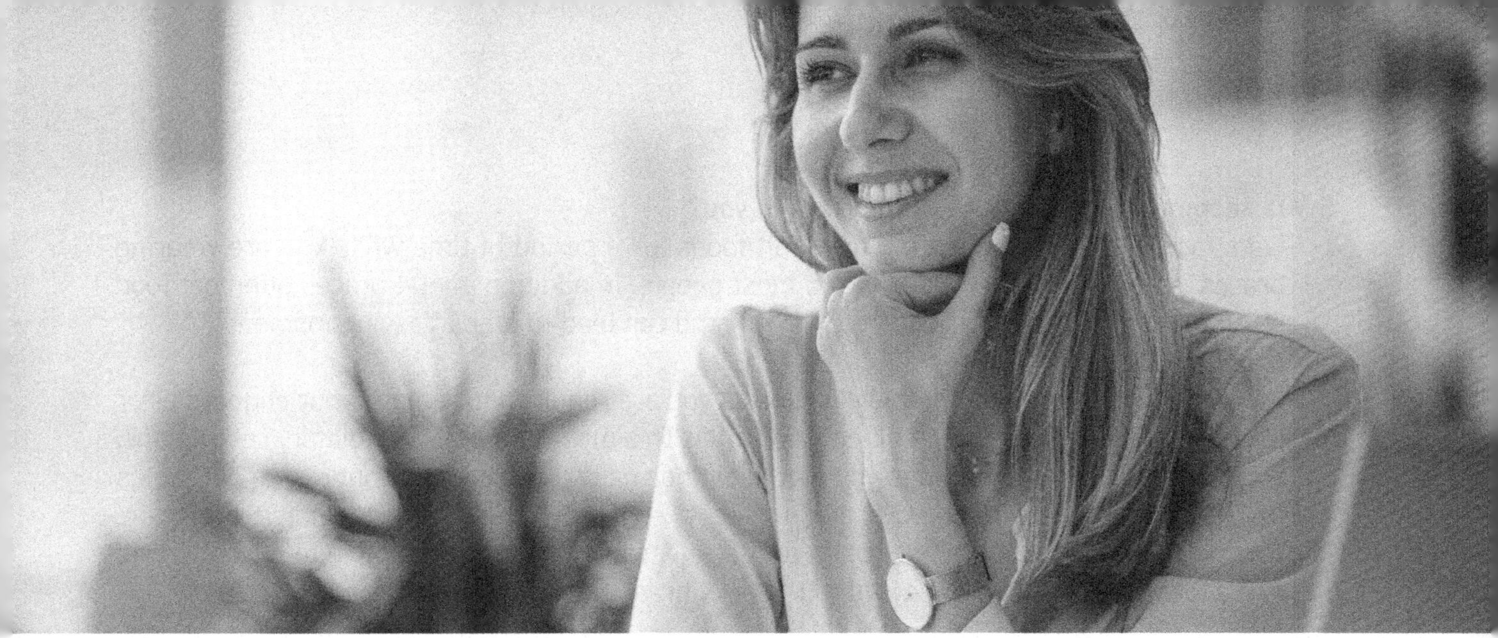

3. **Are you looking for the best value in the least amount of time?**
   In this book we have discussed that one of the benefits of Invisalign is that your treatment time is generally a little shorter than treatment with traditional braces, and it requires less visits to the orthodontist or dentist's office. There are also additional treatments that you can pursue in order to accelerate the process further and cut your treatment time by 30-40% in some cases.

   This means that you will achieve your ideal smile faster, but it also means that your overall cost will be comparable with metal braces. This makes Invisalign the ideal choice for patients who want to get the most efficient treatment and the best value at the same time.

4. **Do you have a special event coming up?**
   If you have a milestone birthday event which you will be celebrating in a grand fashion, or if you are getting married in the near future - you will naturally want to look your best for the occasion - and for the photos that will be taken to commemorate it!

   Invisalign is a great solution for taking care of any issues with your smile that makes it less than picture perfect. With adequate planning time, you can have your treatment completed way before the event or milestone, which will have you smiling on more ways than one!

5. **Is keeping your regular diet important to you?**
   Let's face it - the idea of eating only soft foods for a period of time while you are wearing braces is not one that is appealing to most people. In addition, metal braces often get food stuck in them that can be difficult to get out and can lead to embarrassing moments.

   Invisalign eliminates both of these issues as you are required to remove your aligners prior to eating or drinking anything other than water. This means you have no dietary restrictions, so you can eat the same things you would eat normally. You can also continue to eat things that are strictly prohibited with metal braces, such as popcorn, hard candies, and gum. This benefit is one that patients often appreciate, since it is less disruptive to their lifestyle and allows you to enjoy a treat without fear of breaking brackets or wires.

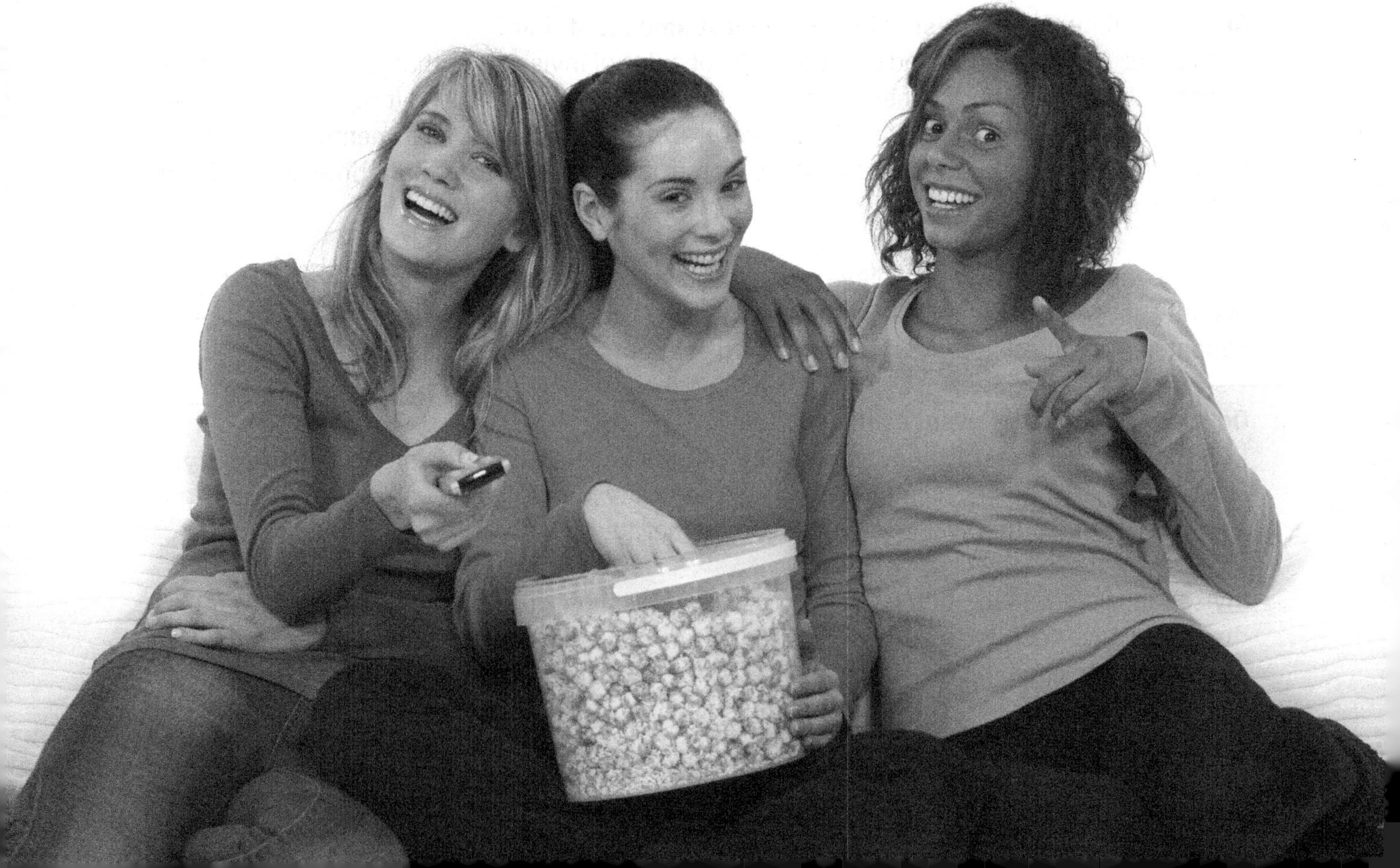

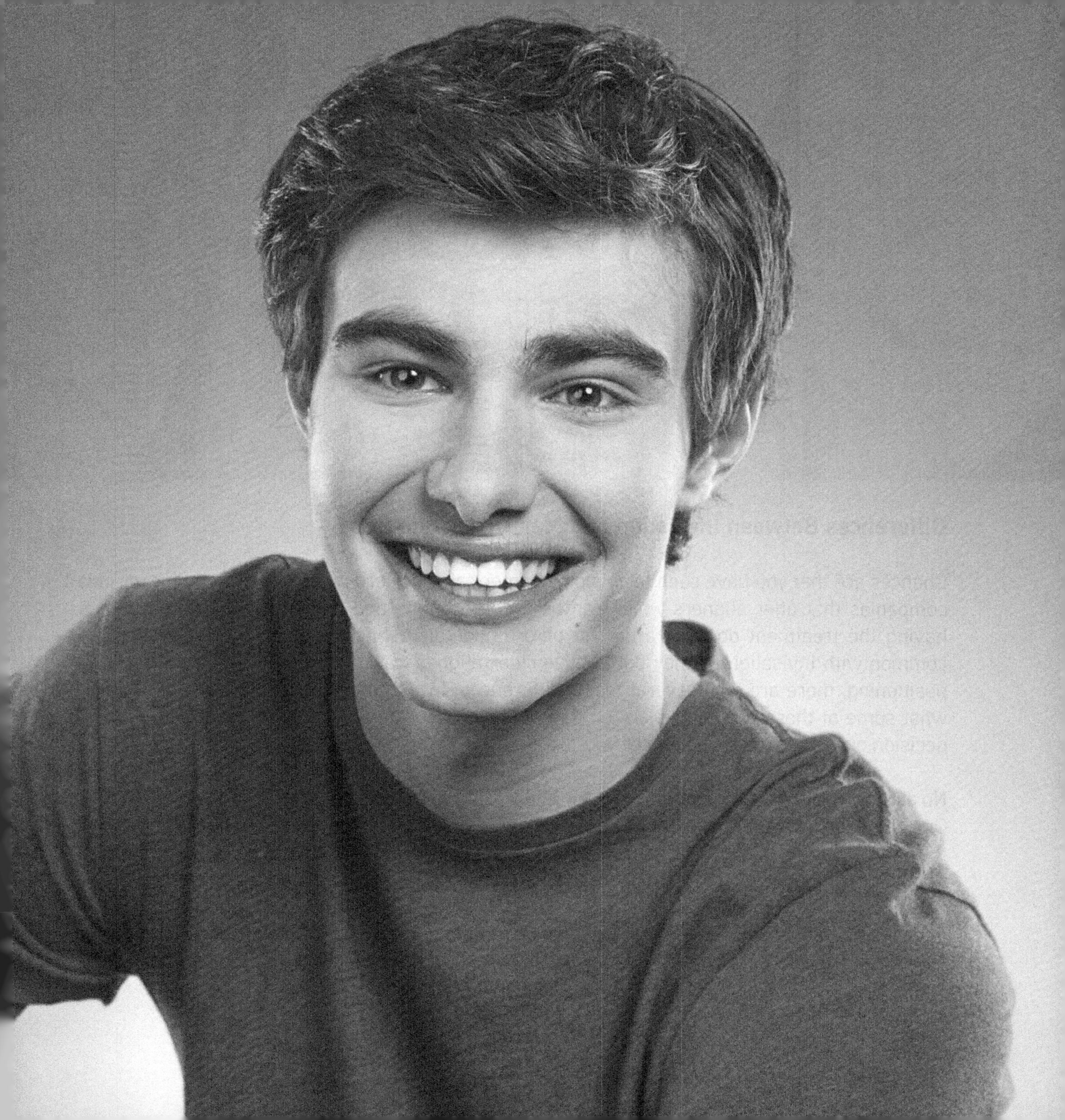

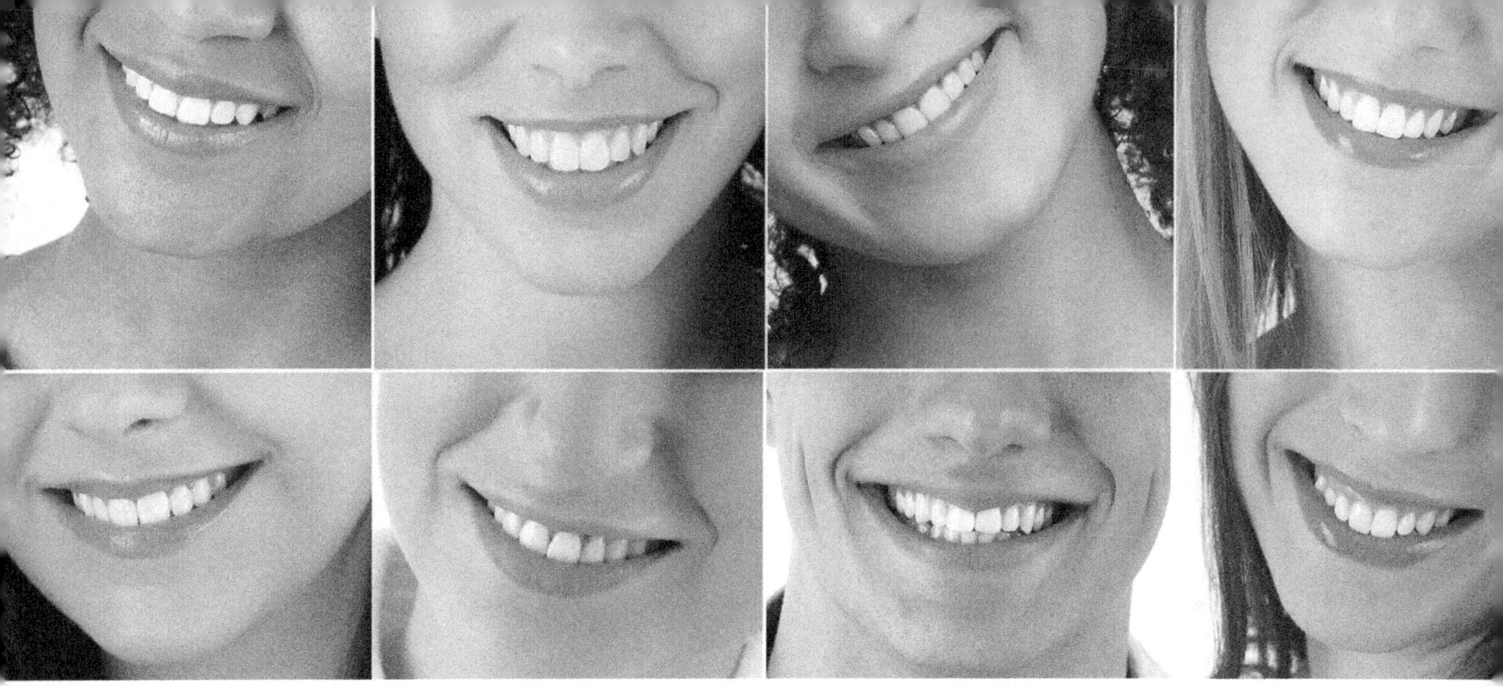

Differences Between Invisalign and Mail Order Aligners

Chances are that you have seen television commercials or heard radio ads recently for various companies that offer aligners which can be ordered online and mailed to your home versus having the treatment done by a dentist or orthodontist. While these services have a lot in common with Invisalign as they both utilize clear aligner trays to shift your teeth into proper positioning, there are also several major differences. In the following section, we will outline what some of these differences are so that you can understand and evaluate each to make a decision on which would be best for you.

No access to a dentist at your disposal for addressing questions and concerns
One of the largest differences between mail order aligners and Invisalign is in the way that your treatment plan is created and delivered. While Invisalign treatment is done by visiting your dentist or orthodontist's office, mail order aligners rely on virtual communication only.

People who hate going to the dentist may be thrilled to not have to go into an office to get their new set of trays, but there are also downsides to this. In the event that something goes wrong with one of your aligner trays or you misplace one, an Invisalign patient can simply contact your doctor's office for assistance or to obtain a replacement if one is needed. With mail order aligners, you rely on calls to support and virtual chat for support, which can take longer to resolve an issue.

Your treatment plan is not created by a person that you know
Since Invisalign treatment is provided by your doctor's office, you establish a rapport with both the doctor and their staff. Your personal dentist knows you and your teeth. They also know your medical and dental history, and they work with you to develop a treatment plan that is created specifically for you. There is a level of comfort associated with that personal touch which is simply not possible with a product that you order online.

While mail order aligners do have a team of licensed dental professionals, the dentist or orthodontist that your case is assigned to is part of a network of affiliated doctors across the country. You are not able to contact this person, therefore you are not able to ask questions about any particular concerns you may have.

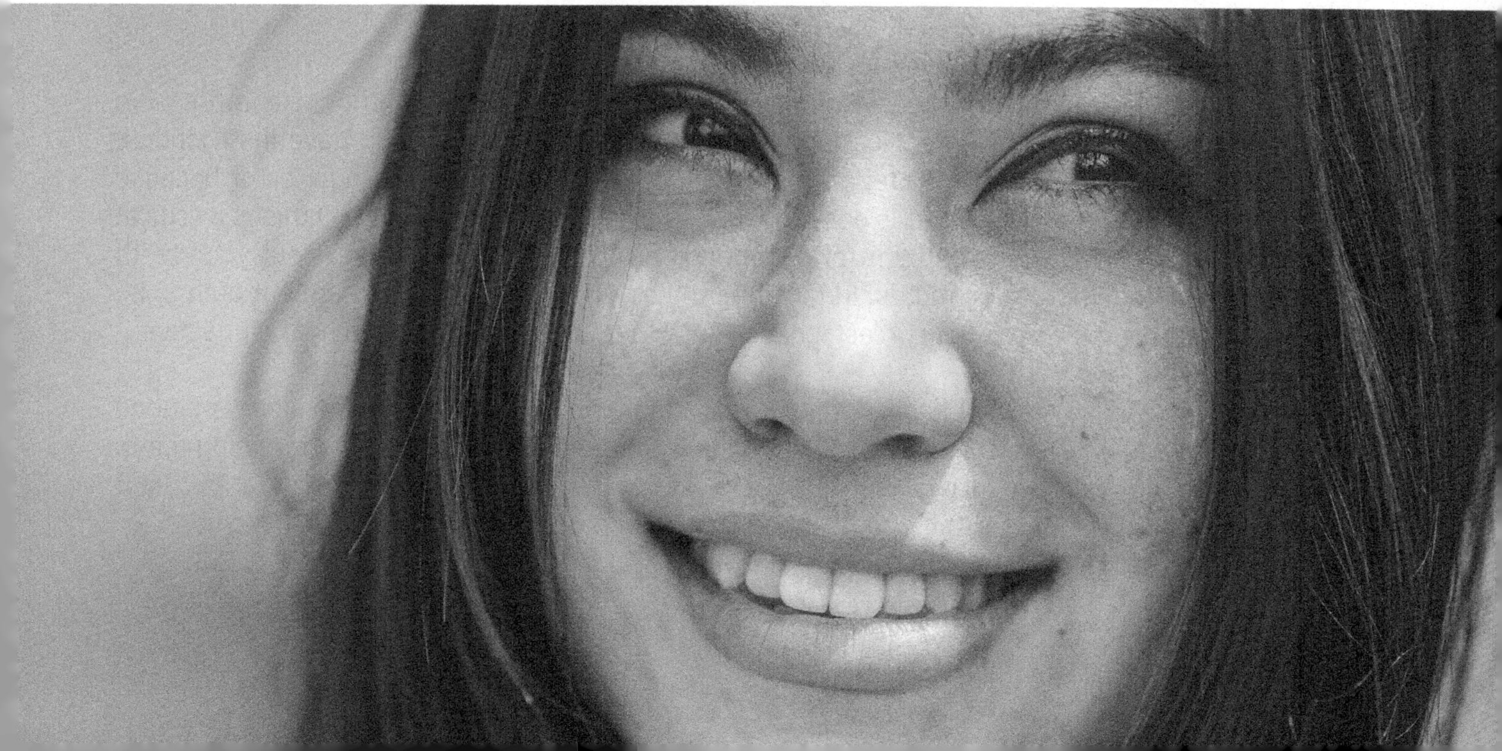

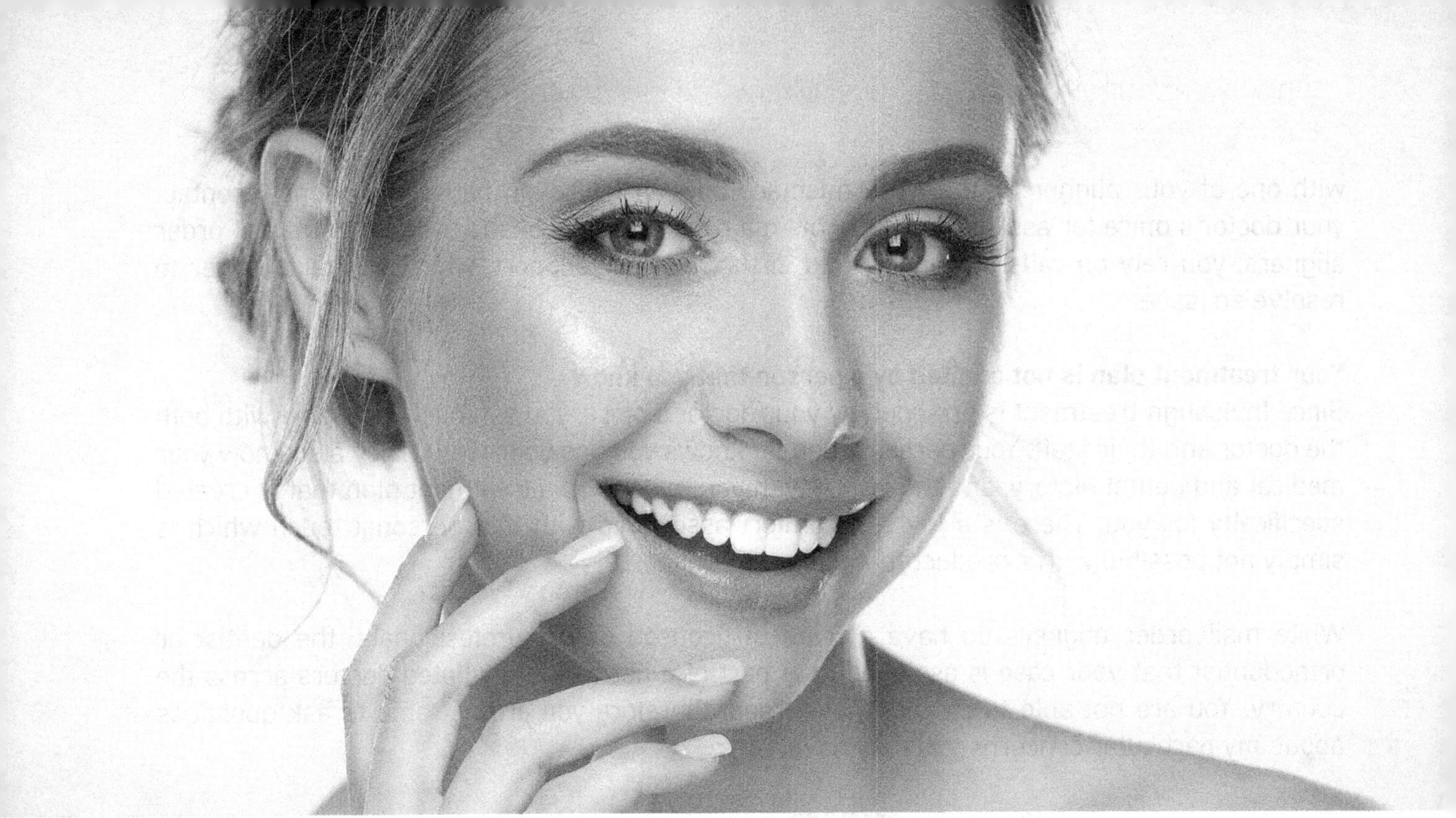

Dental impressions have less room for error with Invisalign

One of the trickiest parts of mail order aligners is that patients are required to take impression molds of their teeth themselves. Most companies that provide aligners do have instructional videos on how make impressions step by step, however, there is always room for error because the patient is not a professional. It is easy to make an improper impression, and this is a critical step, because much of the treatment plan depends on what can be learned about your teeth from studying the impression molds. In fact, it is the only real way for the treatment plan to be formulated. If the molds are not correct, chances are that your results will be not be effective.

With Invisalign, you have the peace of mind knowing that your scans and impressions are done by a professional who is certified in dispensing the treatment, and an expert in examining teeth. It is your best option for ensuring that your are receiving the plan and the aligners that best suit your needs and the smile that you hope to accomplish at the end.

Mail order aligners can only treat basic straightening cases

While Invisalign can treat a wide variety of situations where a patient wishes to have their teeth straightened, mail order aligners can really only be used for teeth alignment issues that are pretty basic. This is fine for patients who meet that criteria, however, patients who need more advanced care such as bite alignment and other issues will be denied the ability to receive treatment and will be advised to seek out a dentist or orthodontist.

There is no fine tuning aspect with mail order aligners

For patients that need them, Invisalign uses small tooth-colored attachments to connect with the aligner trays. This is common in complex cases where additional subtle movement is needed to straighten particular teeth, and it is technology that is only available to Invisalign patients.

Mail order aligners do not have this capability, therefore those cases are also advised to seek out a dental professional for their treatment.

Another fine tuning aspect that Invisalign offers over mail order aligners is that there is a trimming process used to custom fit each aligner tray. This provides a better fit, better appearance, and greater level of comfort.

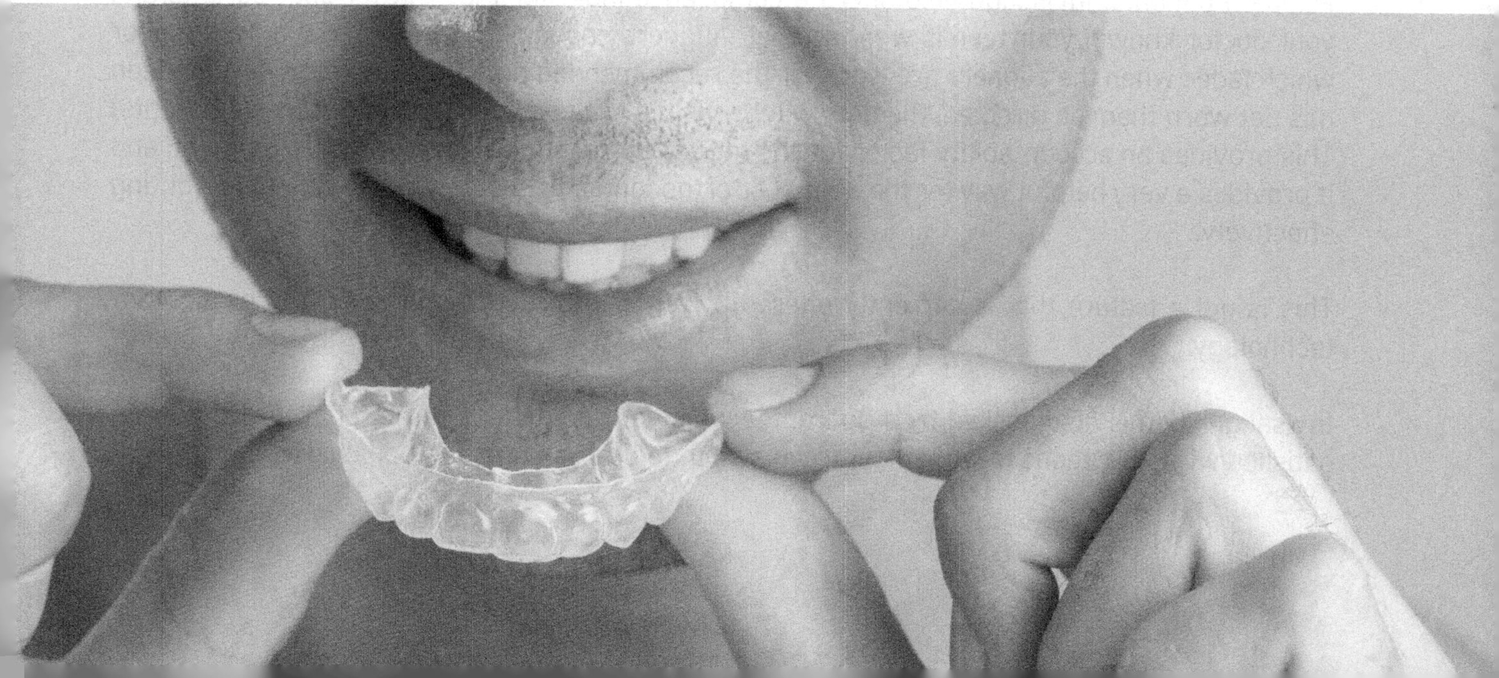

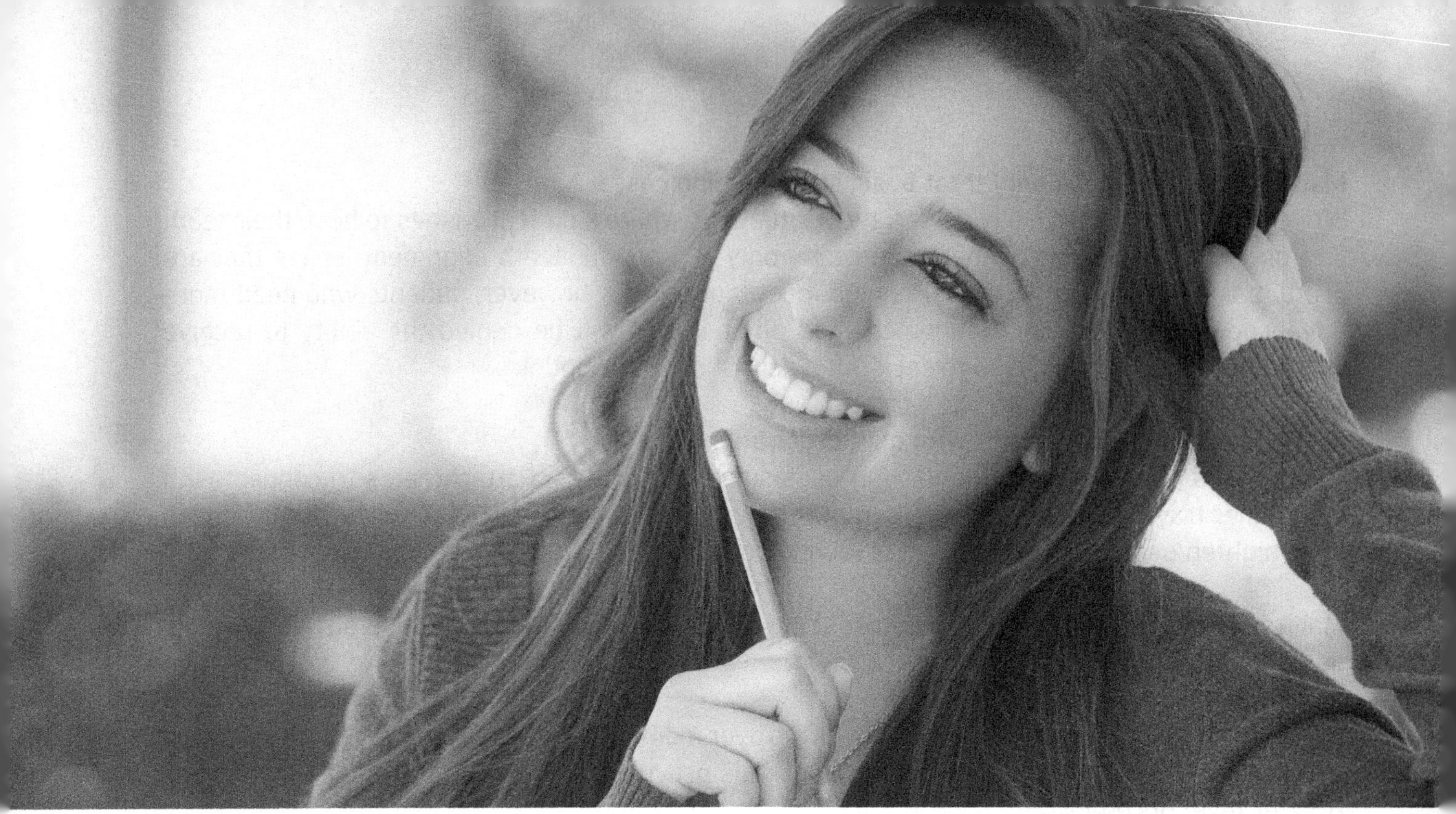

For teen patients, Invisalign also offers a compliance indicator that will let both parents and your doctor know if your teen is wearing their aligners enough. This consists of a blue sensor which fades when the aligners are worn for the recommended period of time each day. If a teen has not worn them as directed, the dots will be visible to the doctor (and to the teen's parents) This provides an accountability factor for the teen to be responsible about their treatment, and it provides a very helpful way for the dentist or orthodontist to ensure that treatment is working effectively.

This is not a feature that is currently offered by any mail order aligners, as it is proprietary technology.

Invisalign Teen is also backed by a guarantee which other aligners do not offer: if you are not satisfied with your teens treatment, you can switch to braces at no additional cost.

There is no accountability or checking in on your treatment with mail order aligners
There are aspects to Invisalign for teens that provides an accountability factor, but let's face it - some adults also need extra help in doing what is best for themselves and their treatment. One of the benefits to have a doctor supervised treatment plan is that your dentist or orthodontist can help you stay on track just by knowing that if you don't follow your plan, you will need to answer for that upon your next visit. Some people just simply need this push to make sure that they received the best results.

However, another huge benefit of being in a treatment plan that is doctor supervised is that when you have regular visits, your dentist can examine your teeth to make sure your treatment is actually working the way that it should. Because conditions regarding your teeth can change even from the time that you begin treatment, this is very helpful in making sure that you get the results in the end that you are expecting - and that you are paying for.

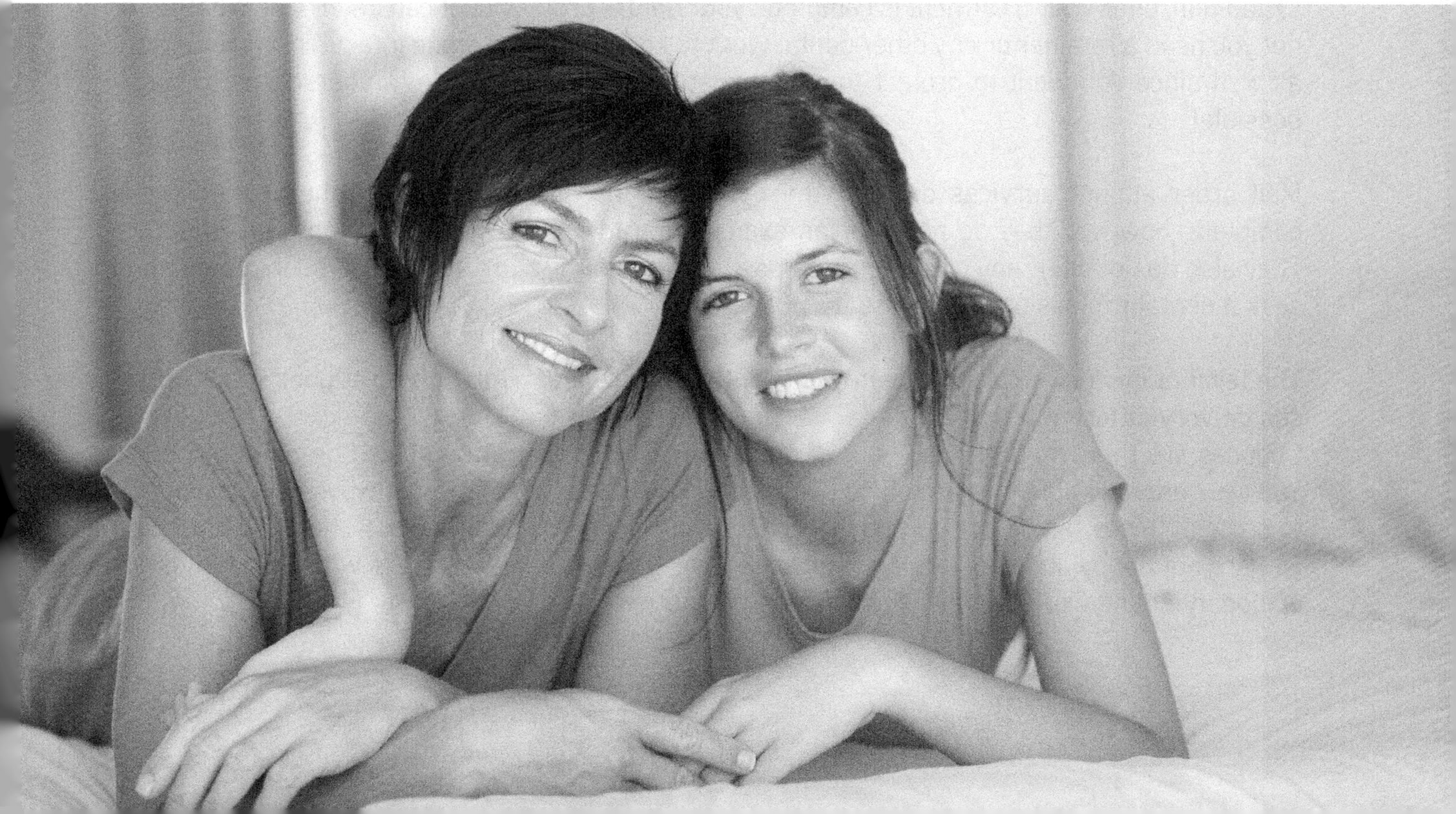

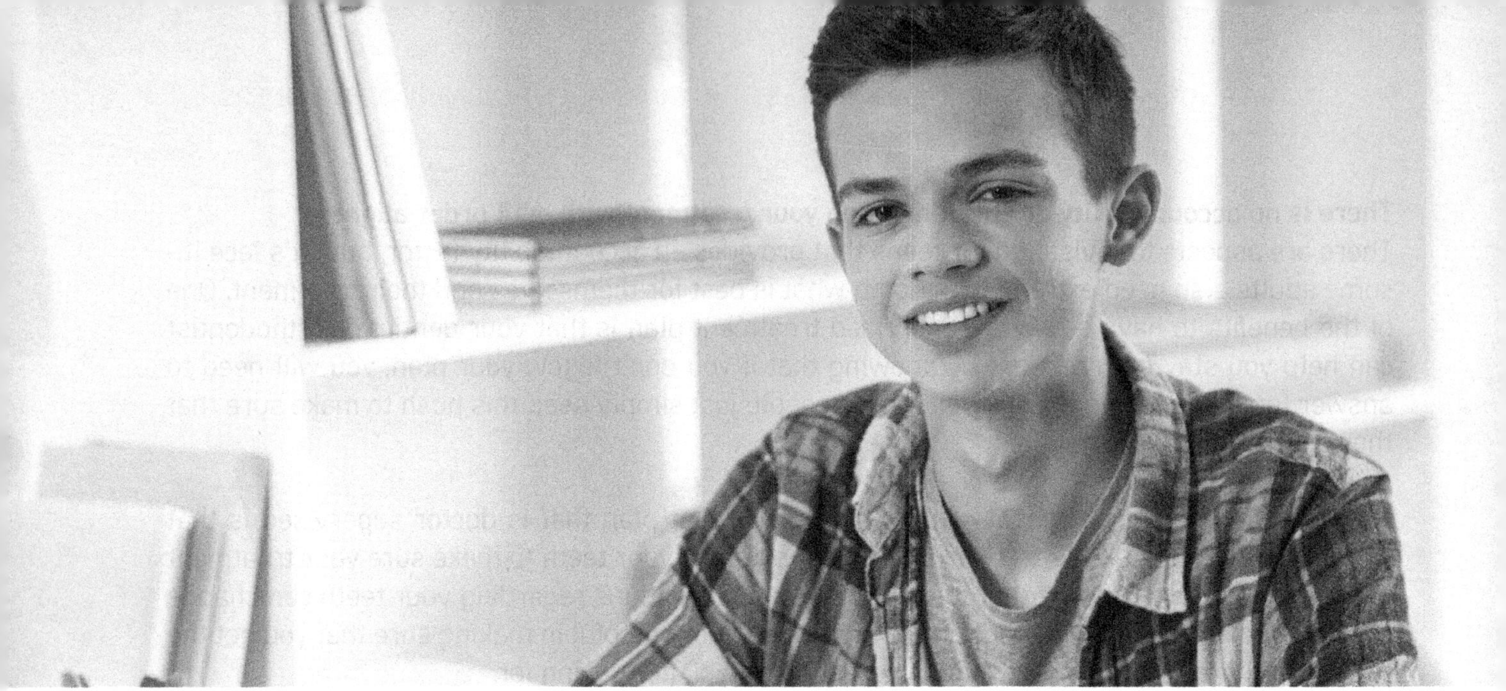

In addition, once your treatment is complete, your dental professional can determine whether or not you need a retainer or any other dental work to keep your new smile intact. This is important as well since you want to protect the investment that you just made in yourself as much as possible!

Mail order aligner services do offer the option to purchase as retainer when treatment is complete, however they do not offer an examination to ensure your treatment was effective. They also do not offer any other services post straightening, and advise that you independently seek a dental professional for these purposes.

The level of customer care between your dentist's office and a mail order aligner's call center can be very different.
Chances are that when you call your dentist's office, you will not be placed on hold for hours. You are generally able to reach a live person quickly and easily, and you always have the option to come in to see the doctor personally to have your concerns addressed. If there is something you are not happy about regarding your treatment, you are able to discuss with your dentist or orthodontist and work together to come to a resolution.

Because this is not possible to do with mail order aligners, patients often complain that customer service in these situations is sub par. Because there is a high demand for this service, long wait times to talk to a service representative can occur. This can be especially frustrating if you are trying to resolve a problem or trying to figure out a logistics issue like a late shipment or incorrect delivery. There is also no real way to alter your treatment plan once it is in motion.

The Bottom Line

The American Dental Association believes that supervision by a licensed dental professional is your best course of action when choosing to undergo any kind of orthodontic treatment. Your teeth are a critical part of your overall health, and using do-it-yourself methods can be not just less effective than those done by a professional, but they run the risk of doing harm if not done correctly. This is why they strongly discourage any treatment plan that does not include comprehensive examinations, x-rays, treatment planning, progress evaluations and other assessments. Mail order orthodontics cannot offer this level of care, therefore it is recommended that you consult with a certified, trained professional for best results.

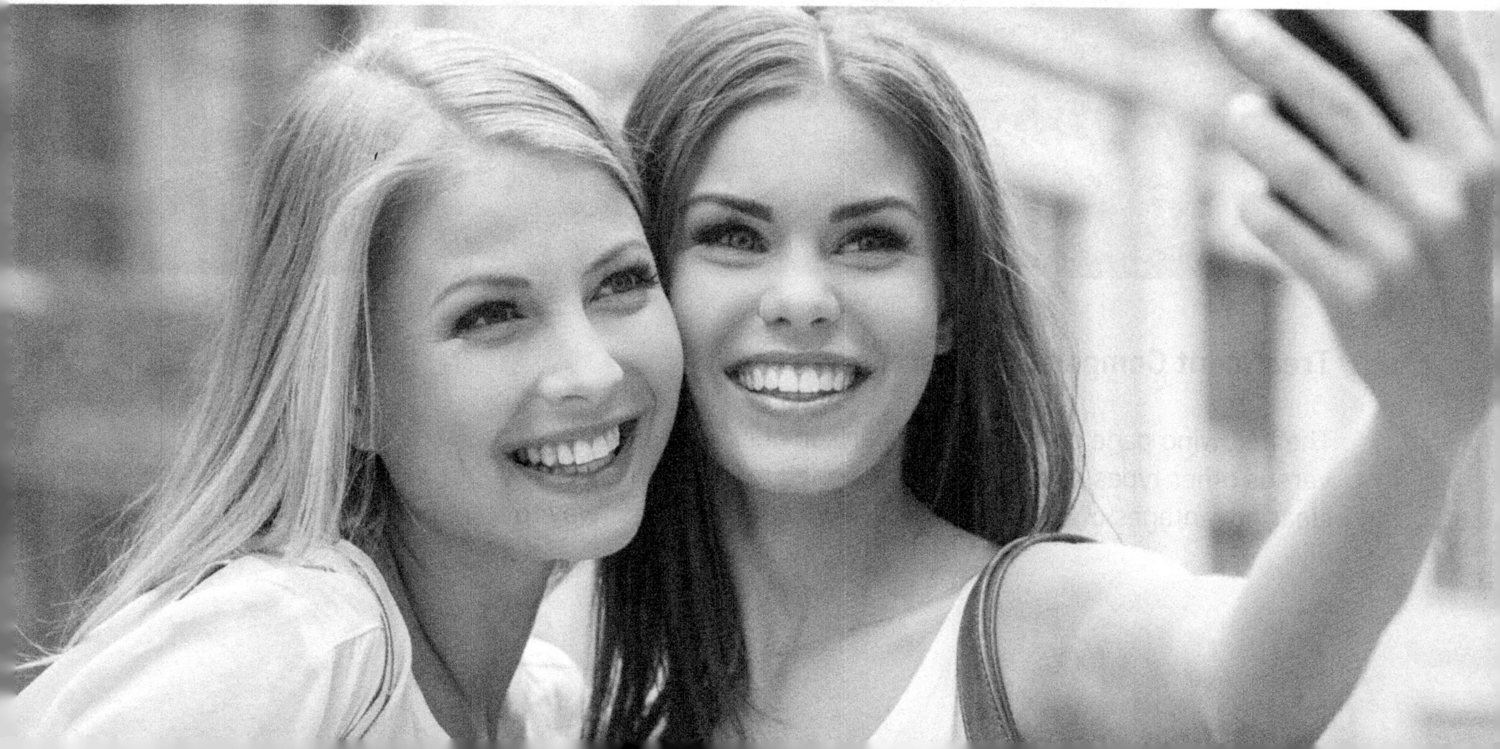

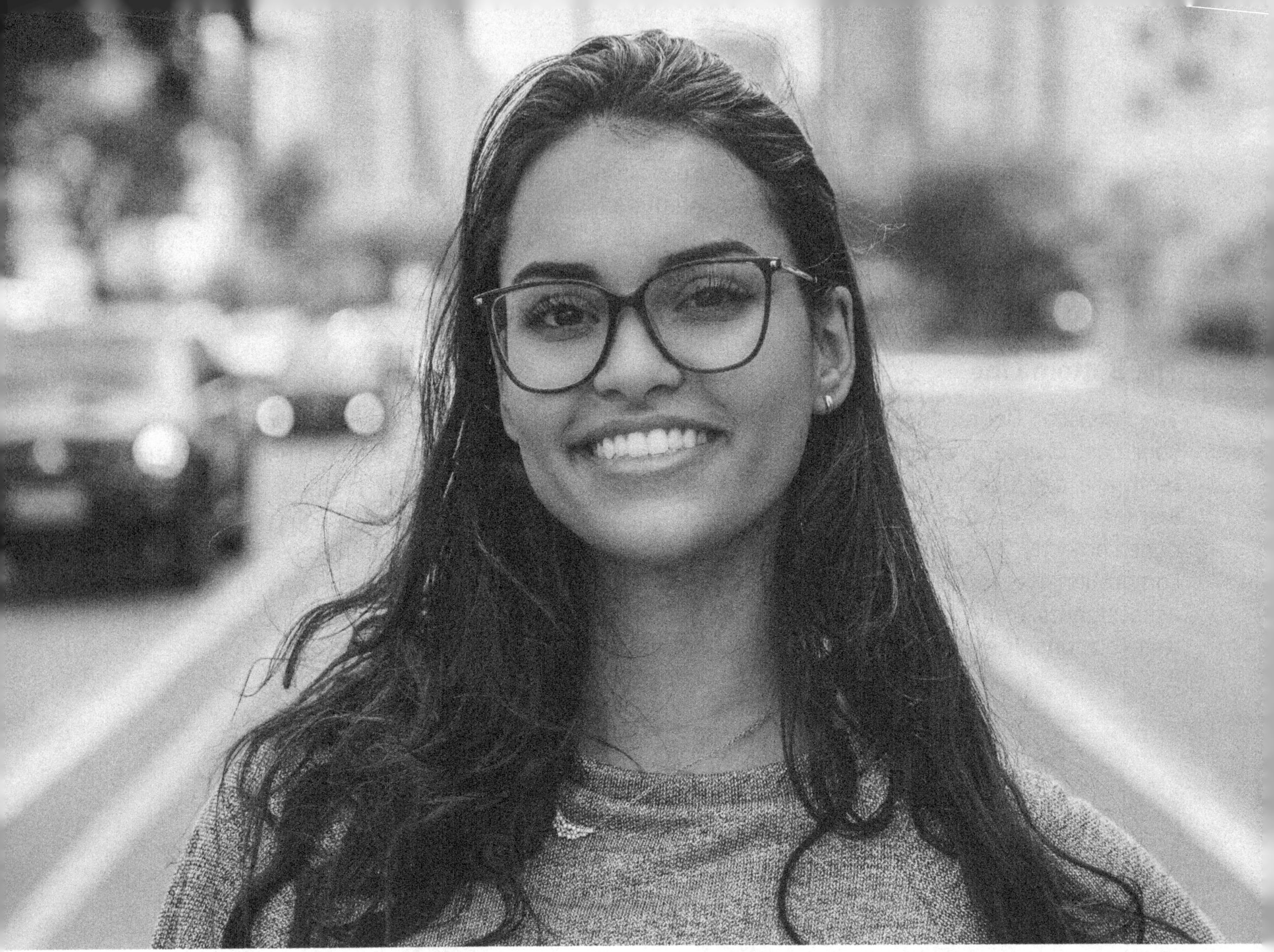

Treatment Comparison Chart

The following page contains a comparison chart that illustrates the benefits of Invisalign versus other types of braces. It is designed to give you an at-a-glance reference for what the clear advantages of Invisalign are, and why it is the best way to transform your smile.

Benefits of Invisalign Over Other Clear Aligners

	Invisalign Clear Aligners	Other Clear Aligners	Traditional Braces
Easily removable for eating and drinking	✓	✓	
No emergency visits for broken brackets and wires	✓	✓	
Virtually invisible	✓	✓	
Easily removable for brushing and flossing with ease	✓	✓	
Made from SmartTrack® material for controlled tooth movement	✓		
Made from off the shelf plastic		✓	
Made from traditional metal brackets and wires			✓
Every aligner is trimmed based on each user's gum line for superior comfort & appearance	✓		
Compliance indicator makes is easy to ensure teens are wearing aligners enough	✓		
Covered by many orthodontic plans	✓	✓	✓
Backed by the Invisalign Teen Guarantee: if you're unsatisfied with treatment within the first 6 months, you can switch to braces at no additional cost.	✓		

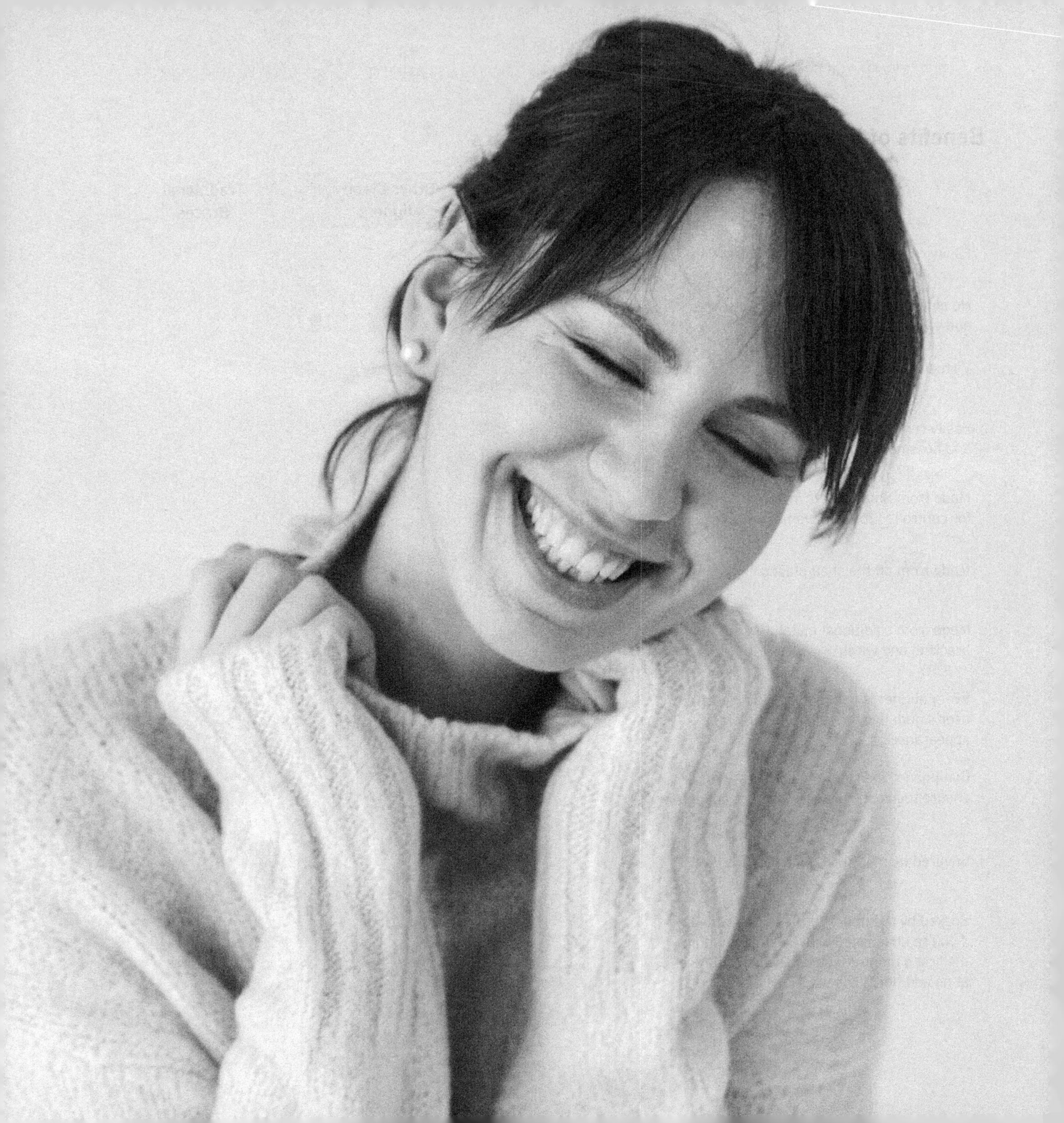

Chapter 4: Cases That Invisalign Corrects

Crowded Teeth

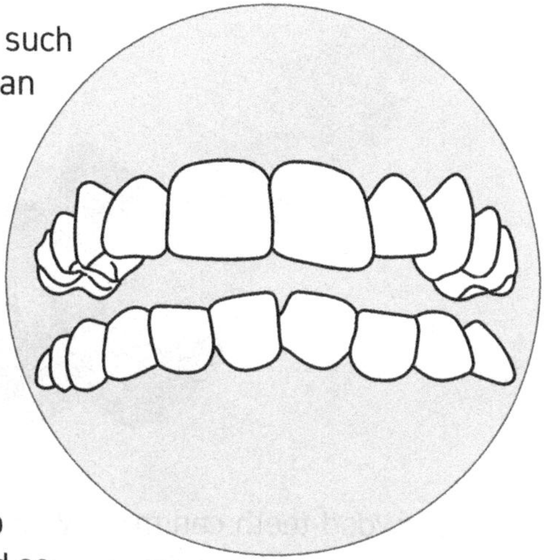

Crowded teeth can be caused by genetics, or by outside issues such as thumb-sucking or extended use of a pacifier as a baby. It can also occur when a child loses their baby teeth early and before their adult teeth are ready to completely grow in. Because adult teeth grow into a spot where the baby version of it previously was, having the previous tooth come out early can cause the adult tooth to drift in the gums. This can result in those teeth shifting, and at times they do that in a space where there is not adequate room for them.

While most adults get a maximum of thirty-two teeth in their lifetime, there are some people who are born with or develop extra teeth. This can cause you to run out of space in your jaw and as a result, your teeth start pressing against each other. This movement causes teeth to become crowded and unseated from their natural position and become crooked.

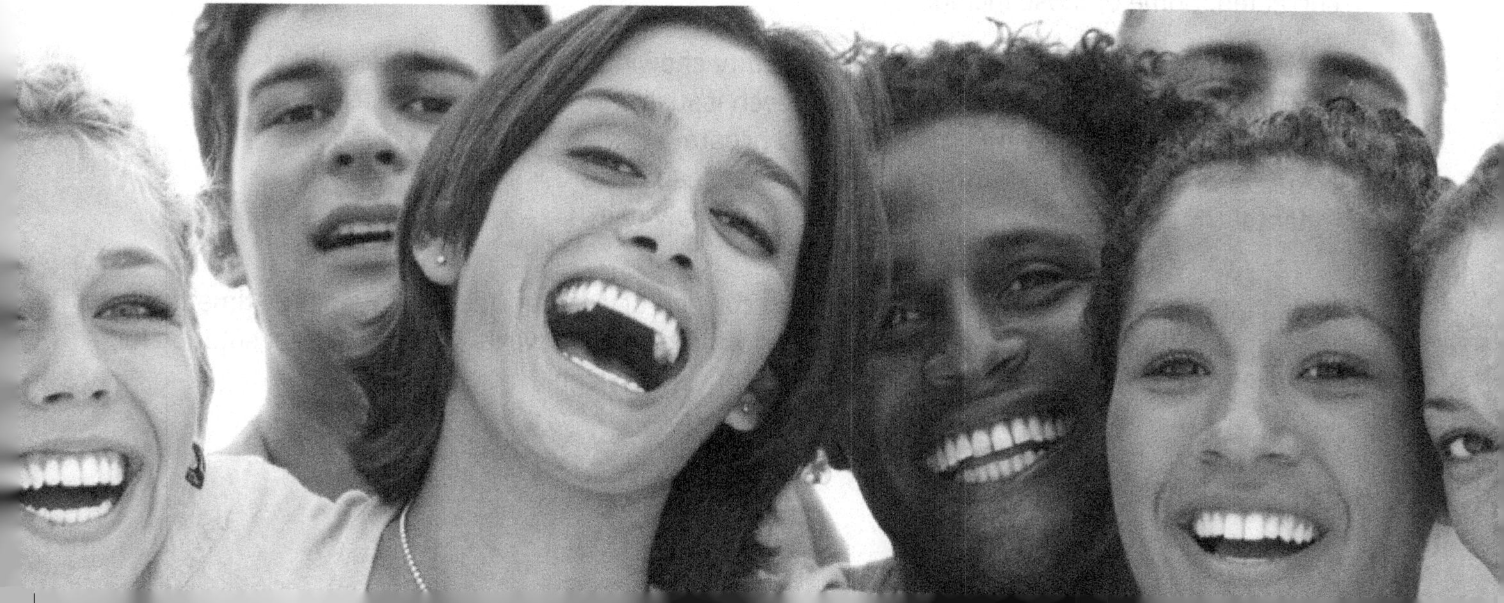

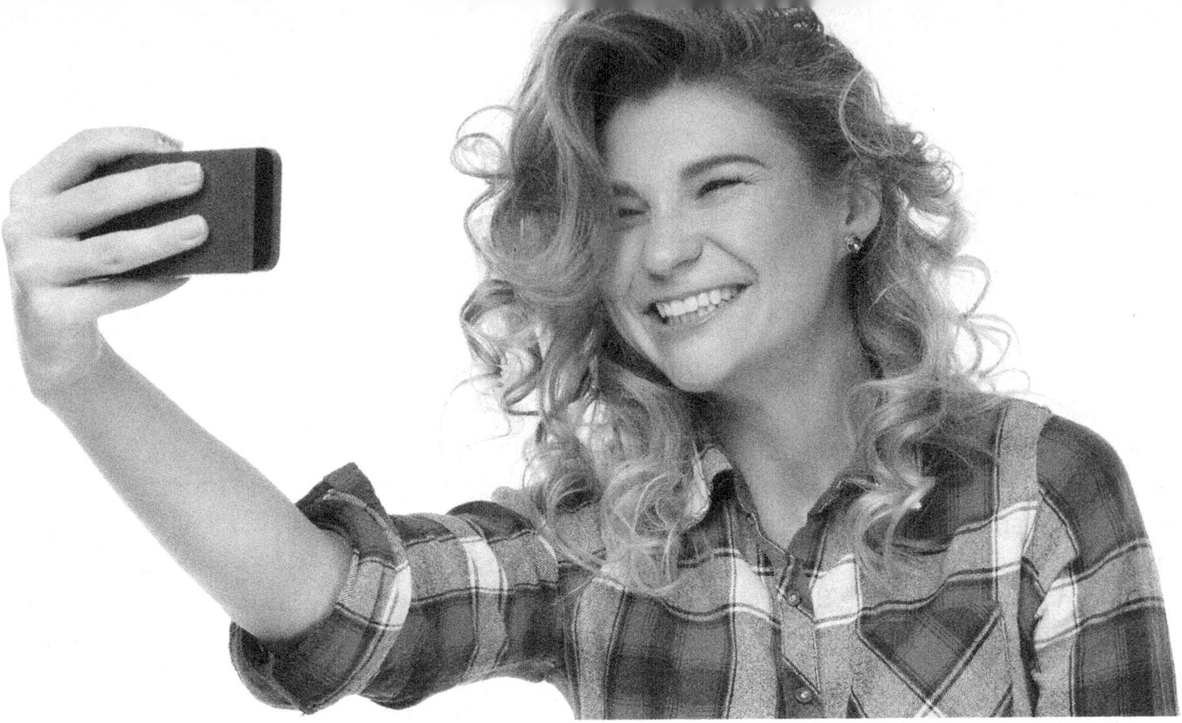

Crowded teeth can make your smile less attractive, and in turn, lower your level of happiness and your self esteem. It can cause teens to face being teased or be made fun of by classmates, and in adults it is not uncommon to see people with crooked teeth consistently hiding their smile.

In addition to aesthetics, there are also health issues that can occur when crowded teeth are not corrected. Some of those include:

- Gum disease
- Malocclusion (bad bite)
- Difficulty with oral hygiene
- Risk of breaking teeth or other dental trauma
- Difficulty chewing
- Speech issues
- Bad breath
- Chronic headaches
- Neck and jaw pain
- Heart disease
- Stroke
- Diabetes

Invisalign can help you correct the issue of crowded or crooked teeth in a smaller time frame than traditional braces, and without the need for brackets and wires. It is the perfect solution for achieving a smile that you'll be proud to show off...at any age!

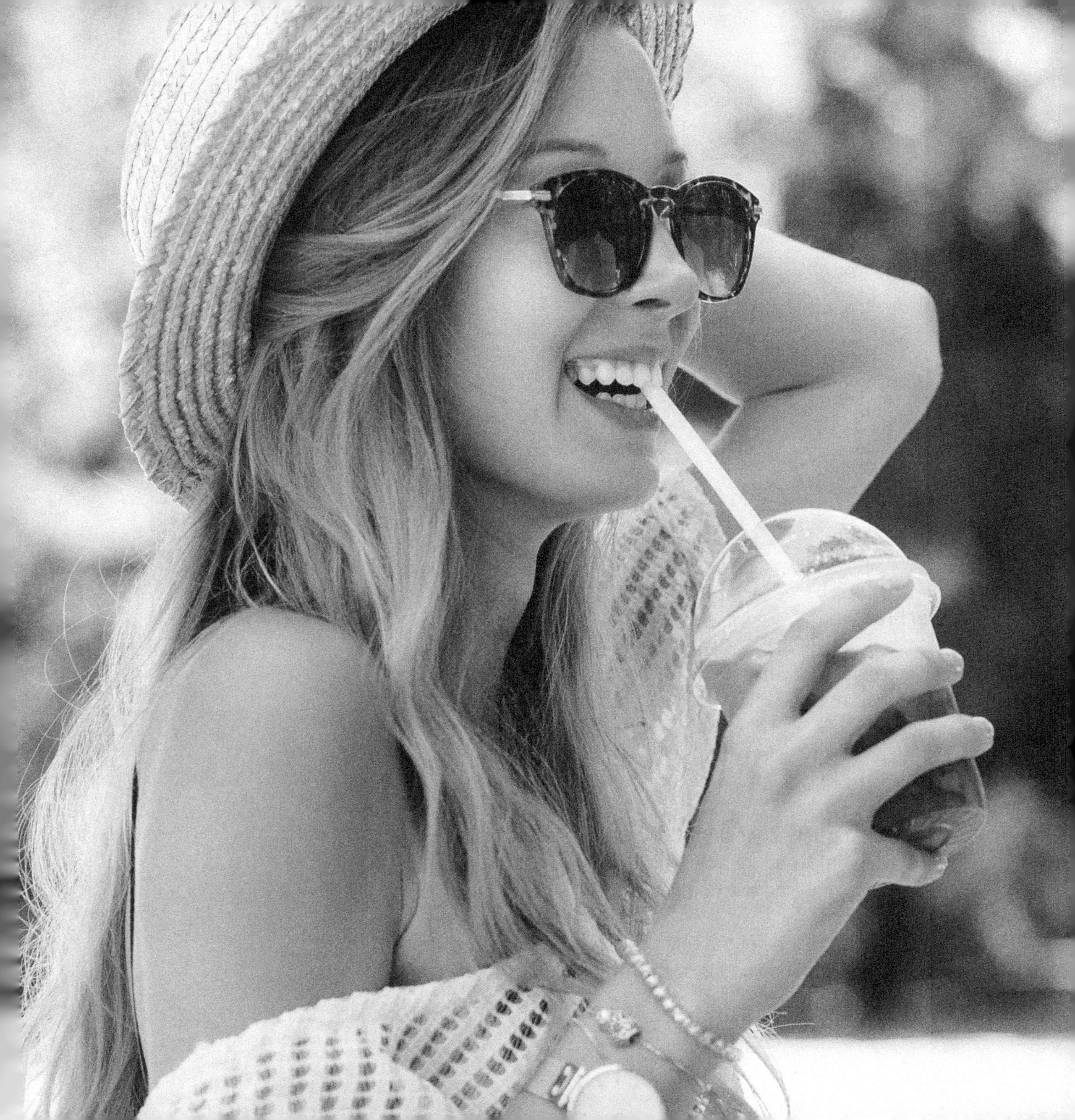

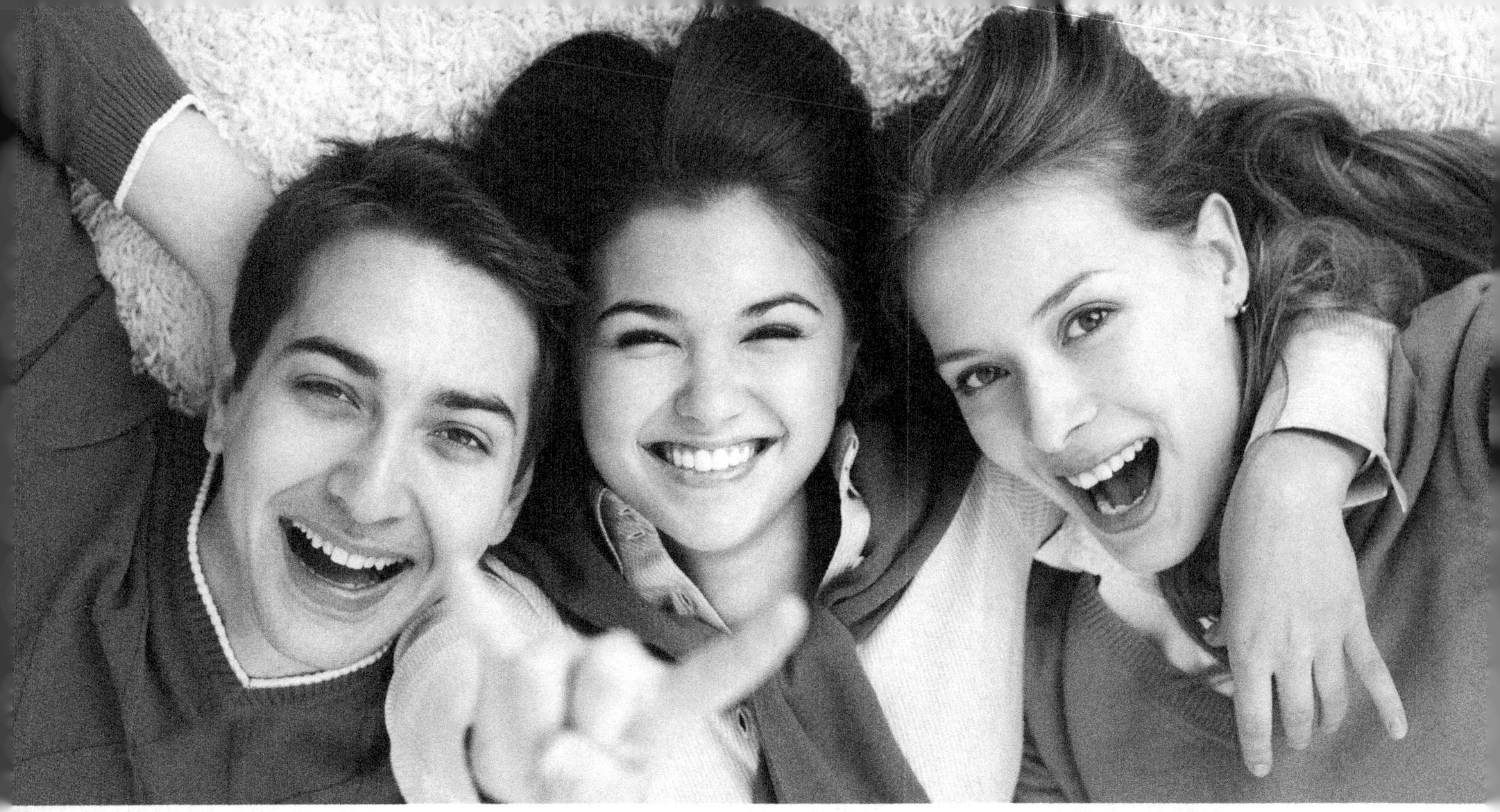

Overbite

This is a condition which occurs when your upper front teeth overlap your lower front teeth. It fairly common and most people have at least a slight overbite. However, when your overbite is too large (commonly referred to as a "deep bite") it can create some health issues if it is not corrected.

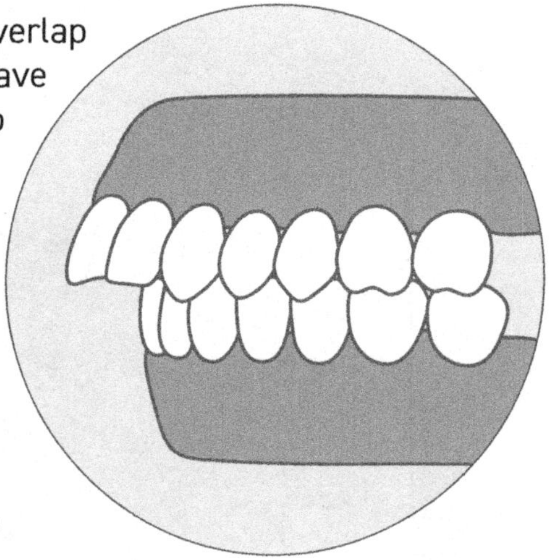

Overbite is largely considered to be an inherited trait, but there are some bad habits which can contribute to the problem - or make an existing one worse.

Thumb sucking is one of the most common and detrimental of these habits. When a child is consistently sucking their thumb, the tongue's thrusting pushes the upper teeth and bone into a more forward position, while the thumb itself pushes their lower teeth back. This then causes the front teeth and jaw to protrude and creates the overbite condition.

Pacifiers and prolonged bottle use after the age of 2 has the same effect as thumb sucking, therefore it can cause the same issue with a child's teeth.

The earlier treatment for this condition can begin, the better as it is a problem which is a frequent target of teasing among children, and it can cause speech impediments that can follow you into adulthood.

Fixing an overbite may be simply a matter of wanting to improve the appearance of your smile, but there are also a number of health issues that can occur if this condition is not corrected, including causing the overbite to get deeper.

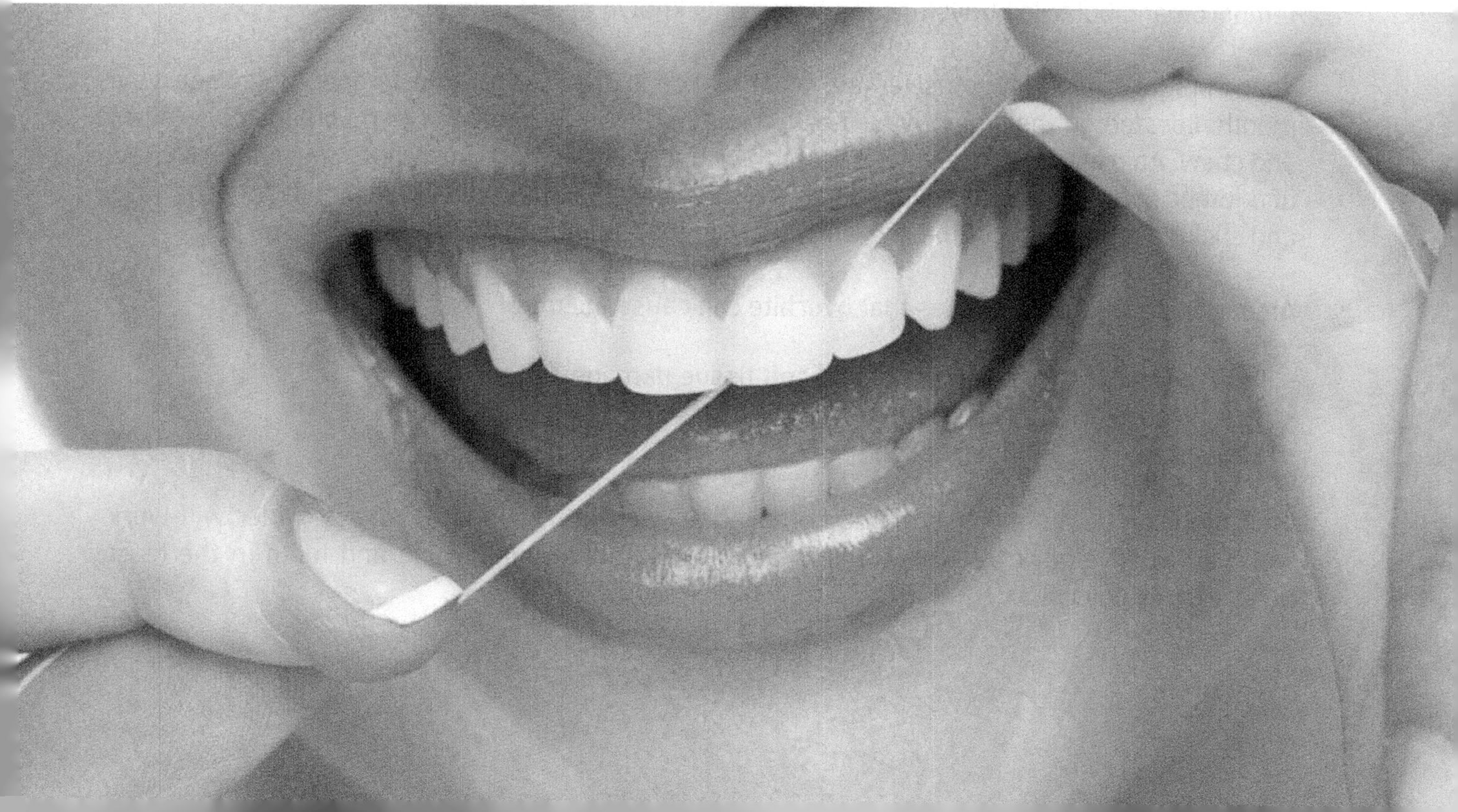

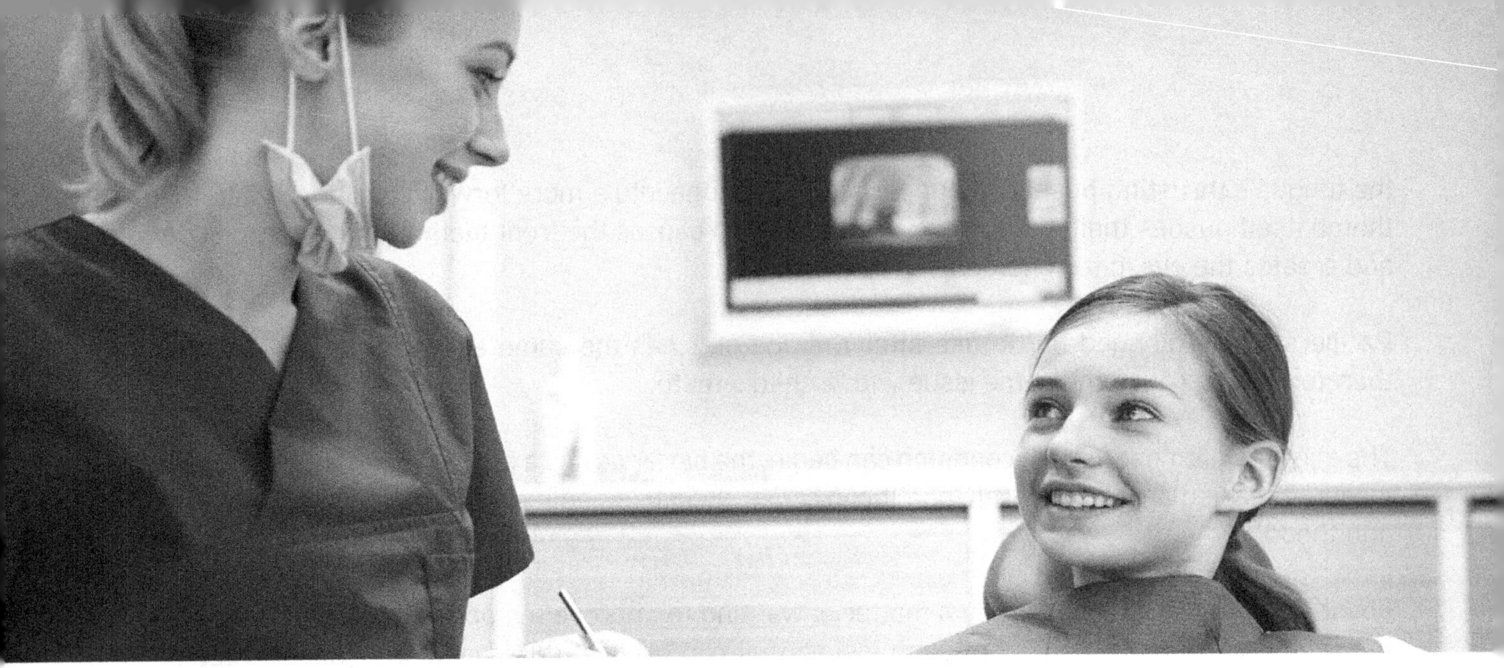

Among one of the one more series condition that can occur from having an overbite is temporomandibular joint dysfunction, commonly known as TMJ disorder.

Your TMJ joints and jaw muscles are what makes it possible for you to open and close your mouth. Located on the side of your head, these parts work together when you speak, swallow and chew. An overbite causes these areas to be overworked more than those muscles in the jaw of another person without this condition. This can cause significant jaw pain, difficulty chewing, and clicking and locking of the jaw, all which can lead to a lot of discomfort.

Among the other health issues that overbite can cause include:

- Tooth decay
- Gum disease
- Headaches
- Risk of tooth and soft tissue damage
- Uneven tooth wear
- Sleep apnea

Invisalign can be an effective method of fixing an overbite/deep bite. Your provider will work with you to develop a treatment plan that will help shift your jawline and teeth in the least invasive way possible.

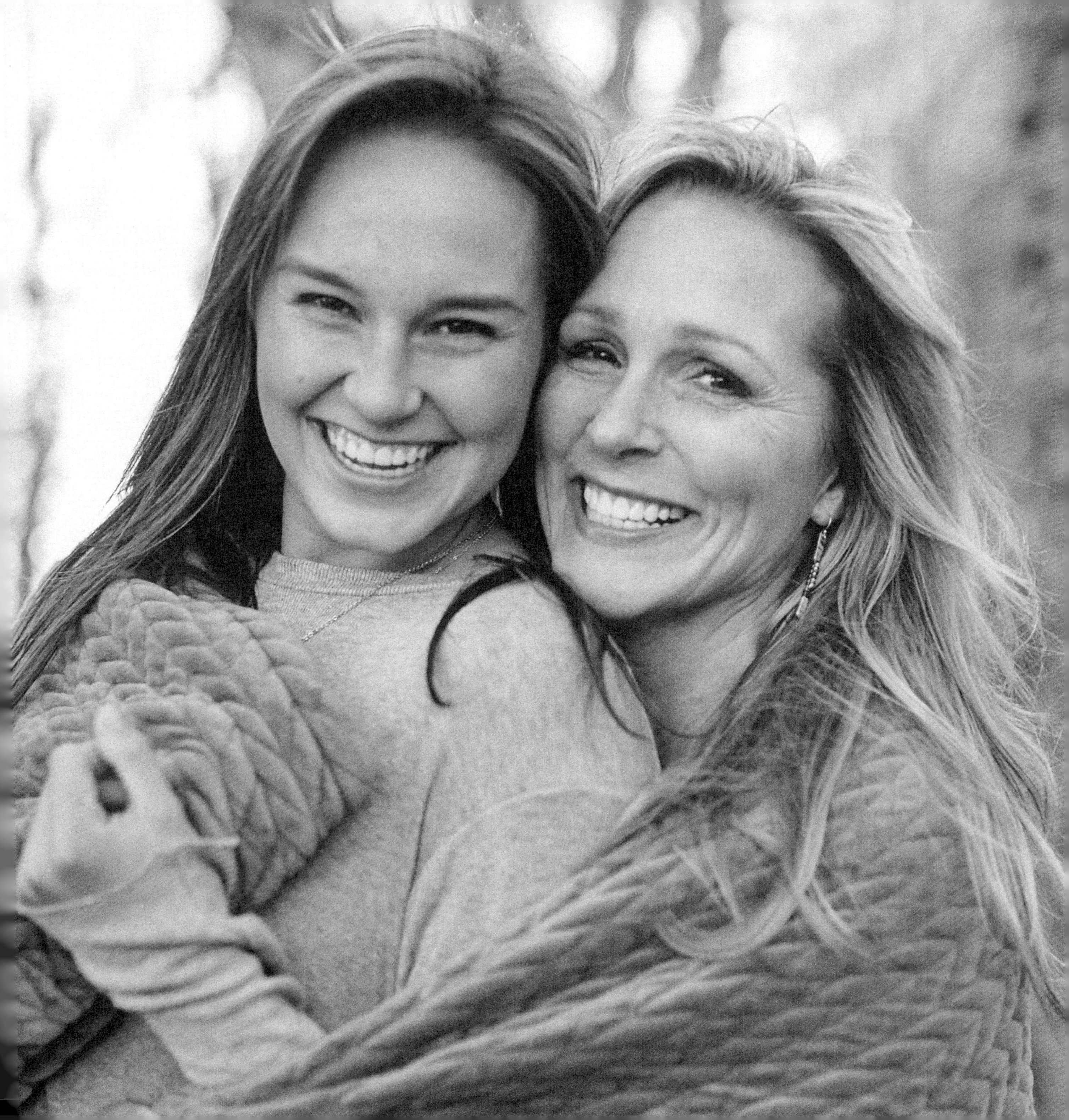

Underbite

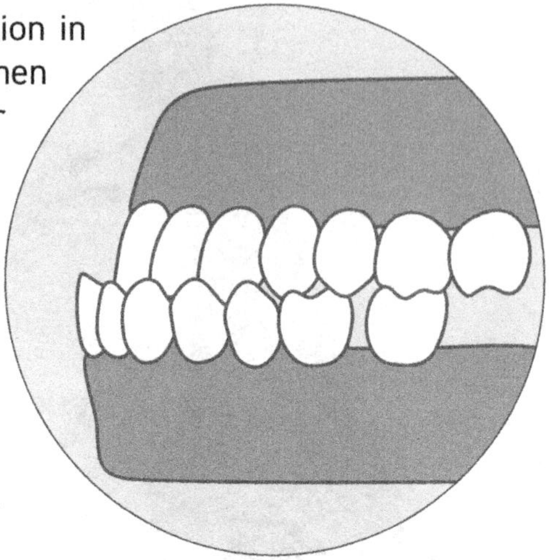

An underbite, also called a Class III malocclusion, is a condition in which your lower front teeth are in front of your upper teeth when your mouth is closed. Normally, your upper teeth cover your bottom teeth slightly - but in a patient with an underbite, the situation is reversed.

Most underbites are genetic - if you had a parent with an underbite, chances are far greater for a child to have one also. Some underbites can also be caused by a bad jaw position (such as your lower jaw being too far forward) or teeth that are in the wrong position. It can also be caused by habits such as thumbsucking or prolonged bottle and pacifier use in young children.

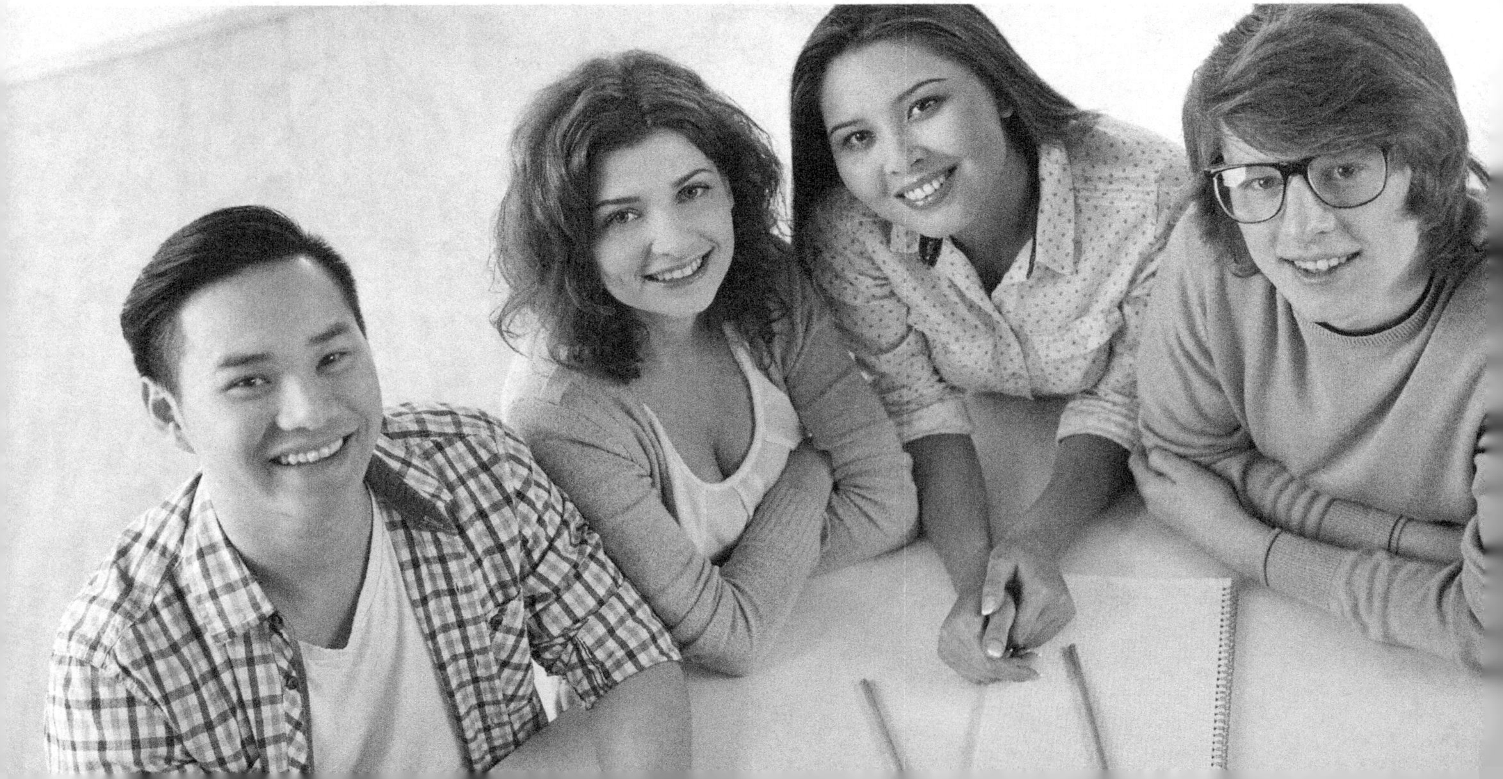

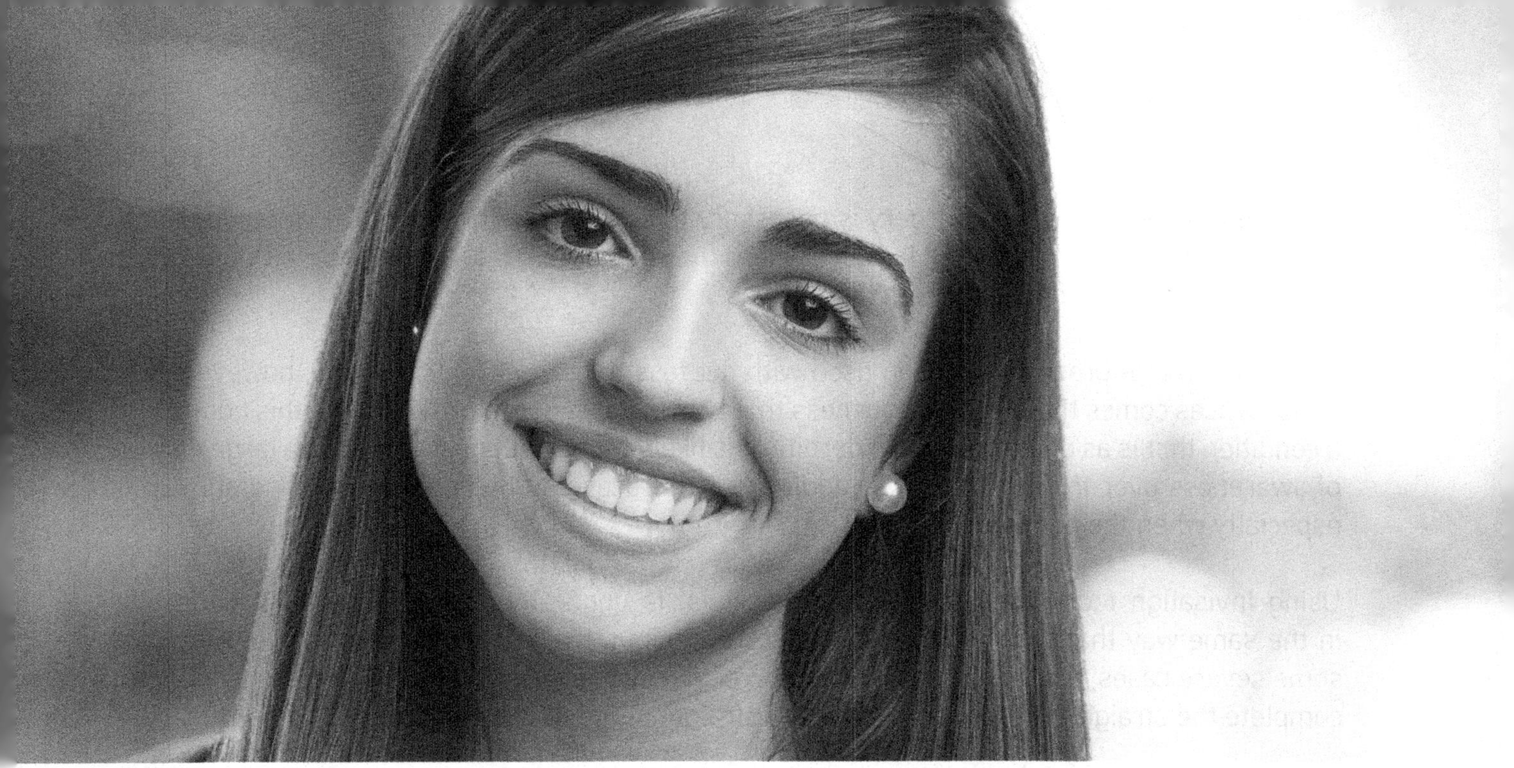

This condition not only looks strange but it can cause some serious health issues. An underbite can inhibit your ability to chew, causing strain in your jaw muscles. It can also make it difficult for you to speak clearly. These can create significant problems not just physically, but socially - therefore it is recommend that a patient who suffers from this condition have it corrected as soon as possible.

Other issues that can be caused by an untreated underbite include:

- Tooth decay due to difficulty in brushing/flossing
- Uneven wearing of your teeth and their enamel
- Temporomandibular Joint Disorder (TMJ)
- Difficulty chewing, which may lead to difficulty digesting

Many years ago, the only way to fix an underbite was for the patient to wear special appliances such as expanders and headgear. These methods, while effective, are uncomfortable and very noticeable - which is why today they are only used when it is absolutely necessary.

In some more severe cases, surgery is necessary to correct the condition. This method is only usually used as a last resort and in cases where the condition is more related to jaw positioning than to issues with a patient's teeth themselves.

Traditional metal braces have been used with success to correct this condition, however, with metal braces comes the self consciousness that we have discussed previously in this book. With a condition that is as obvious as an underbite, it is likely that a patient already has a large degree of awareness over their condition, so adding metal braces can be demoralizing and stigmatic, especially when the patient is a teen.

Using Invisalign technology, a dental professional is generally able to correct an underbite in the same way that traditional metal braces do, minus the stigma and visibility of metal. In some severe cases, a patient can undergo corrective surgery first and then utilize Invisalign to complete the straightening process - and the straight smile that they desire.

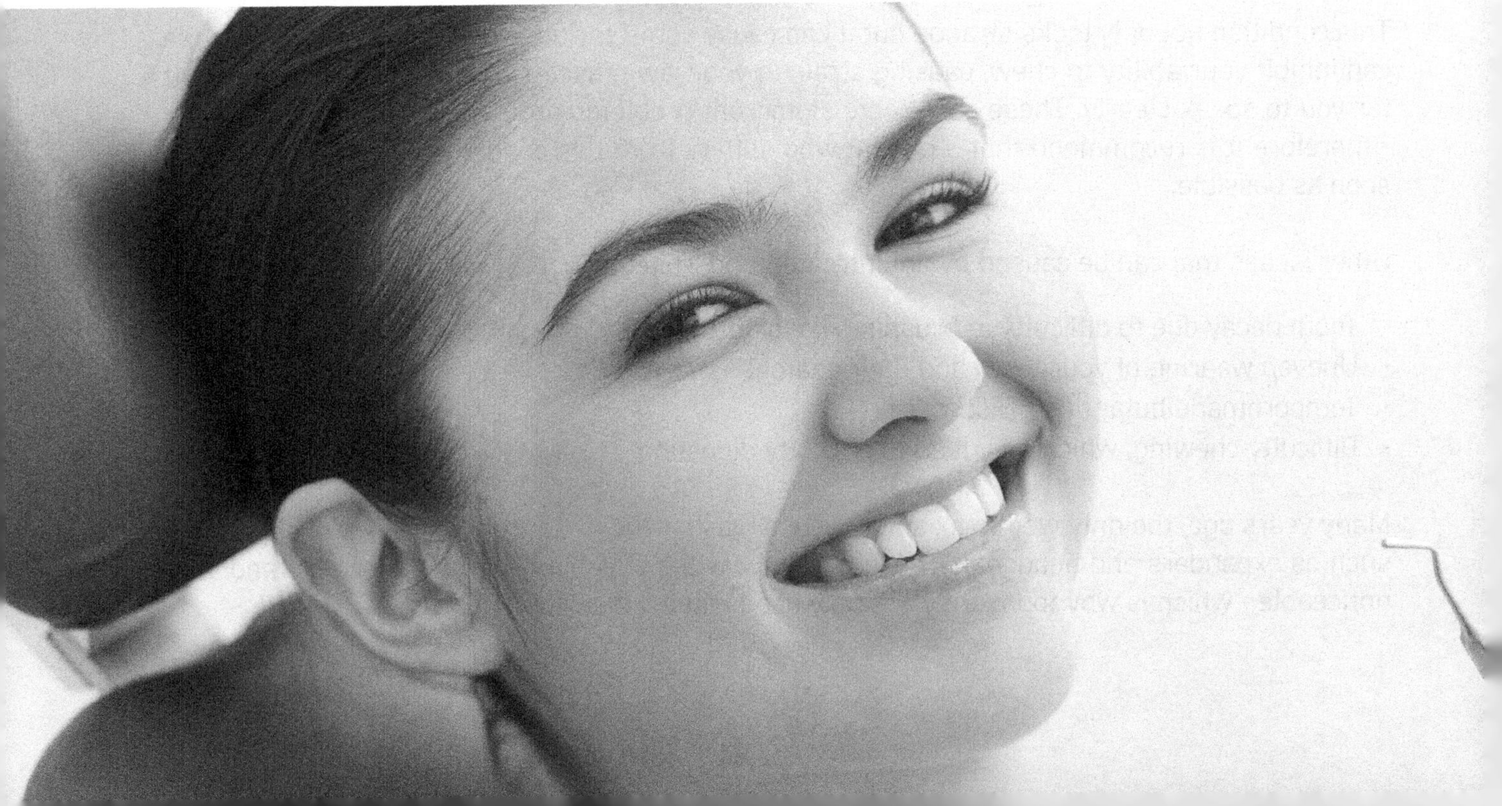

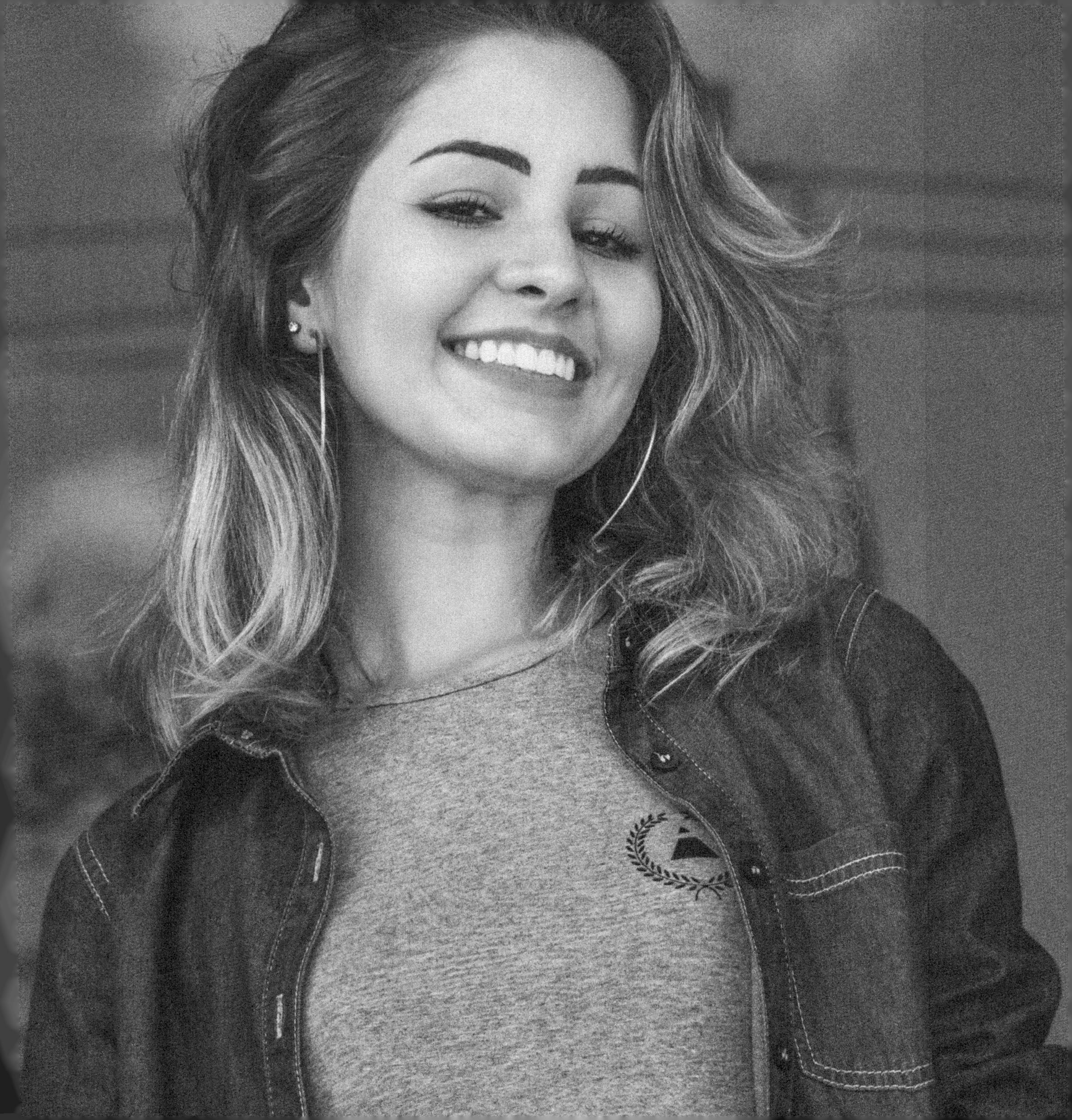

Crossbite

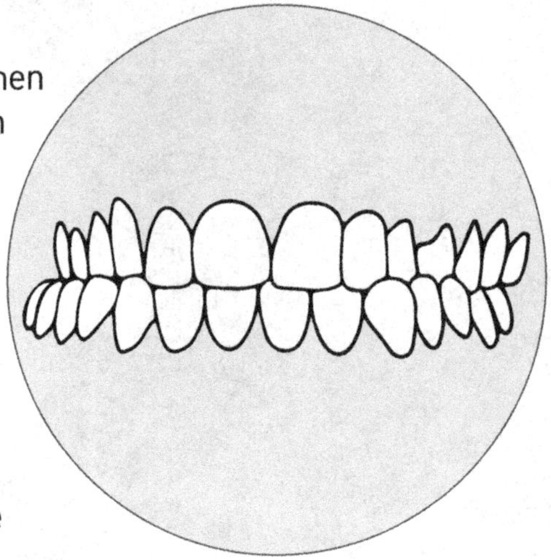

Crossbite is a misalignment of your dental arches. It occurs when some of your upper teeth are seated inside your lower teeth rather than on the outside as they normally would. A misaligned bite of this nature is normally detected in childhood and does not correct itself as adulthood approaches.

It is believed that crossbite is a hereditary condition, however it can also be caused by delayed or abnormal tooth eruption. When baby teeth are lost and adult teeth are delayed in coming in, it can cause the corresponding teeth on the opposite jaw to not meet up with it's counterpart, and that creates the conditions for the crossbite to form.

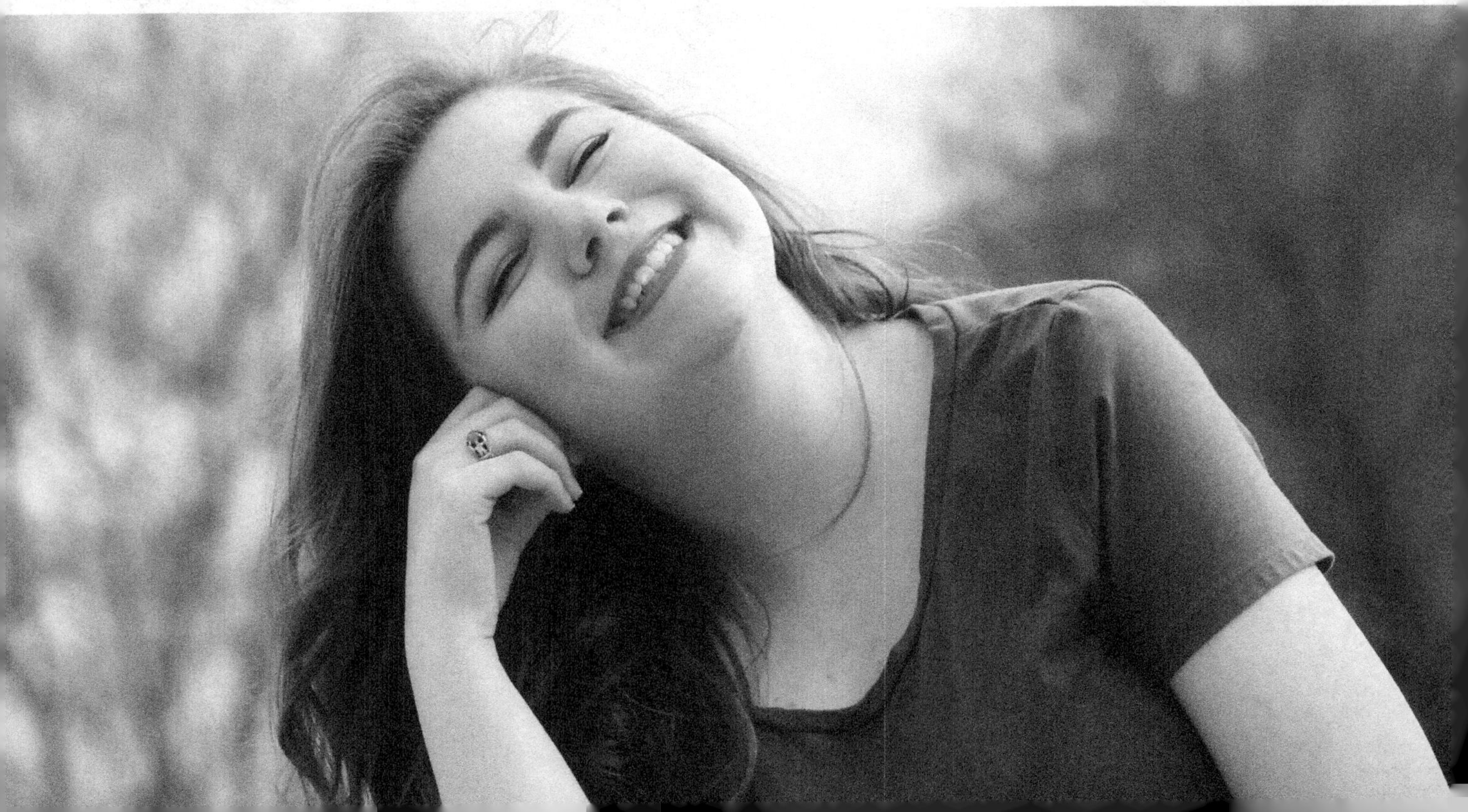

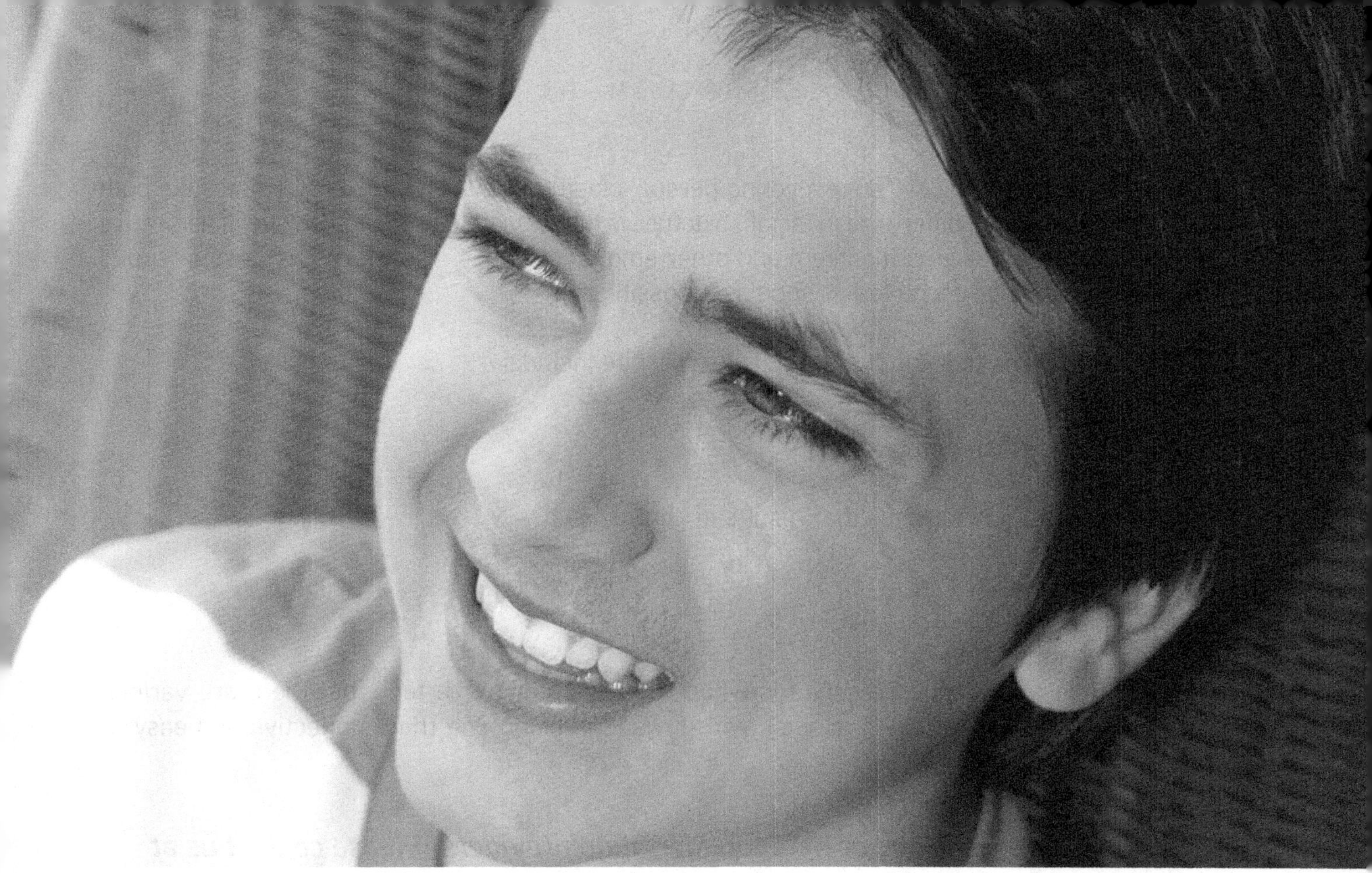

Recent studies have shown that there are several other factors which can cause a crossbite as well, including thumb sucking, prolonged bottle use, and using pacifier after the age of 2. All of these habits push the teeth out of their natural position. Continuing this habit also causes the width of a child's dental palate to be made smaller, deforming the upper bone, which can create a crossbite.

Another factor that has been shown to cause crossbite is mouth breathing. While everyone breathes through their mouth from time to time, some children do this regularly due to enlarged tonsils or other respiratory issues. This can be detrimental to the growth of their jaw, and can create a misalignment that requires correction by a dental procedure.

In addition, a crossbite can cause a young person's face to grow asymmetrically. Because both the crossbite and this difference in facial structure is highly visible to the naked eye, it can cause you to suffer from lower self esteem and other emotional issues. Therefore it is recommended that this condition be corrected as soon as it possible.

Other health issues that can occur due to a crossbite include:

- Tooth decay
- Gum disease and gum receding
- Bone loss
- Stress on the jaw muscles that results in chronic pain
- Neck pain
- Shoulder pain
- Back pain

The best time to correct a crossbite is when you are a child or a teen, but there are various treatments available to adults as well, with Invisalign being one that is effective and easy to implement.

TS Orthodontics is one of NC's top Invisalign providers. Please contact us at 828-254-4602 or visit our website at www.mytsosmile.com to set up your complimentary Smile Assessment.

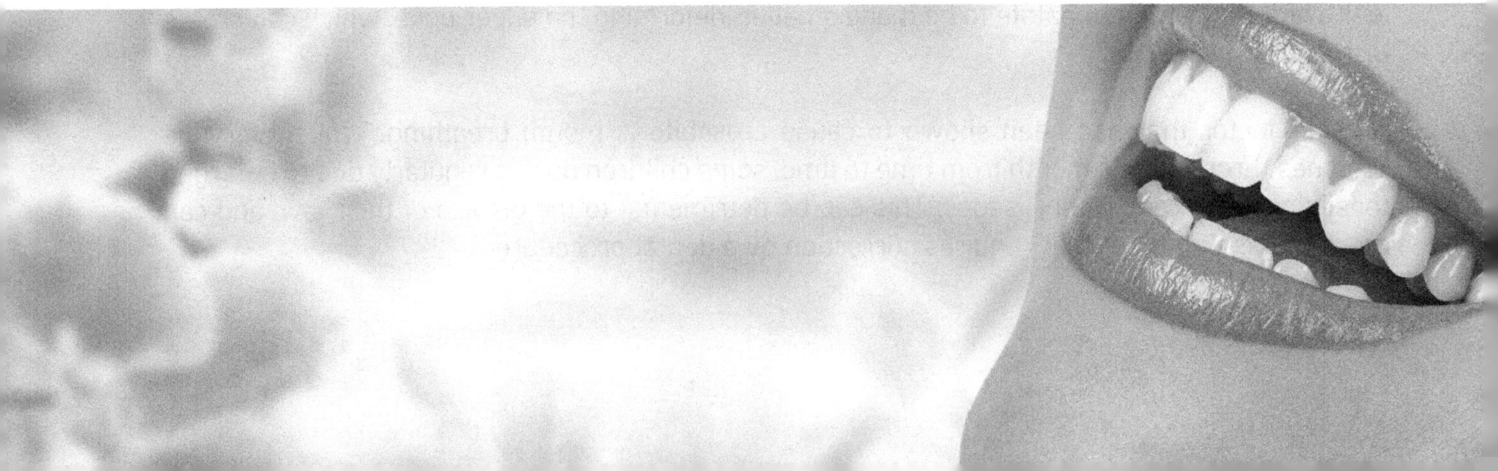

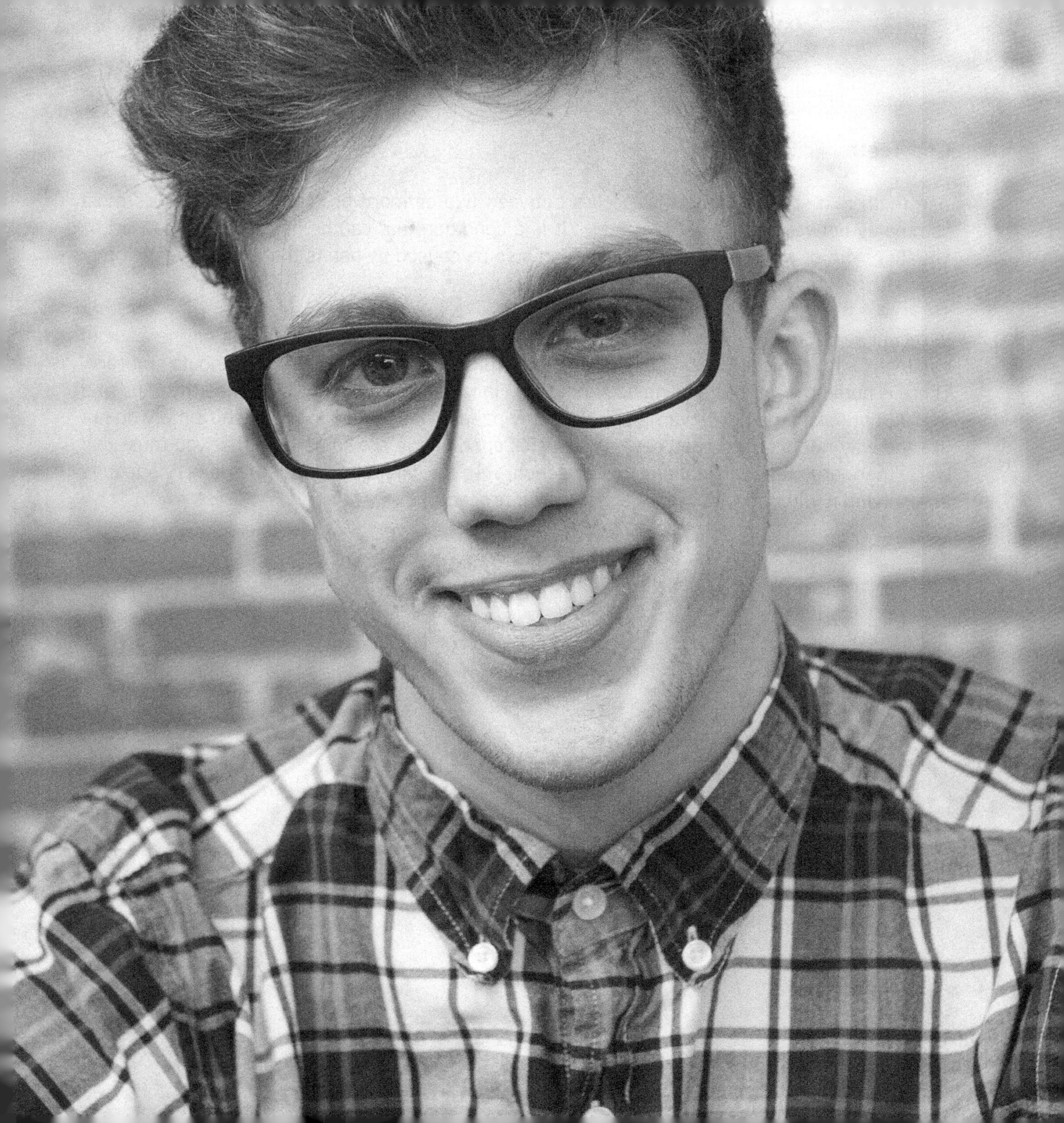

Gap Teeth

Gap teeth is a spacing issue that occurs between two or more of your teeth. It occurs most commonly between your two front teeth. It is a condition that can be hereditary or caused by situations out of your control, however, it can also be caused by habits that children develop at ages where intervention can be difficult.

In recent years, many individuals including celebrities have been shedding light on the issue of gap teeth, with some embracing it as something which is a part of you that you should embrace. There is nothing wrong with being body-positive - in fact, it is encouraged for a healthy mind and overall outlook on life. However, there are many people who have gap teeth who simply do not like the way it looks. The good news is that this condition is not something that you must live with - there are numerous options for correction, with Invisalign being one that is very effective in resolving it without complicated and invasive procedures.

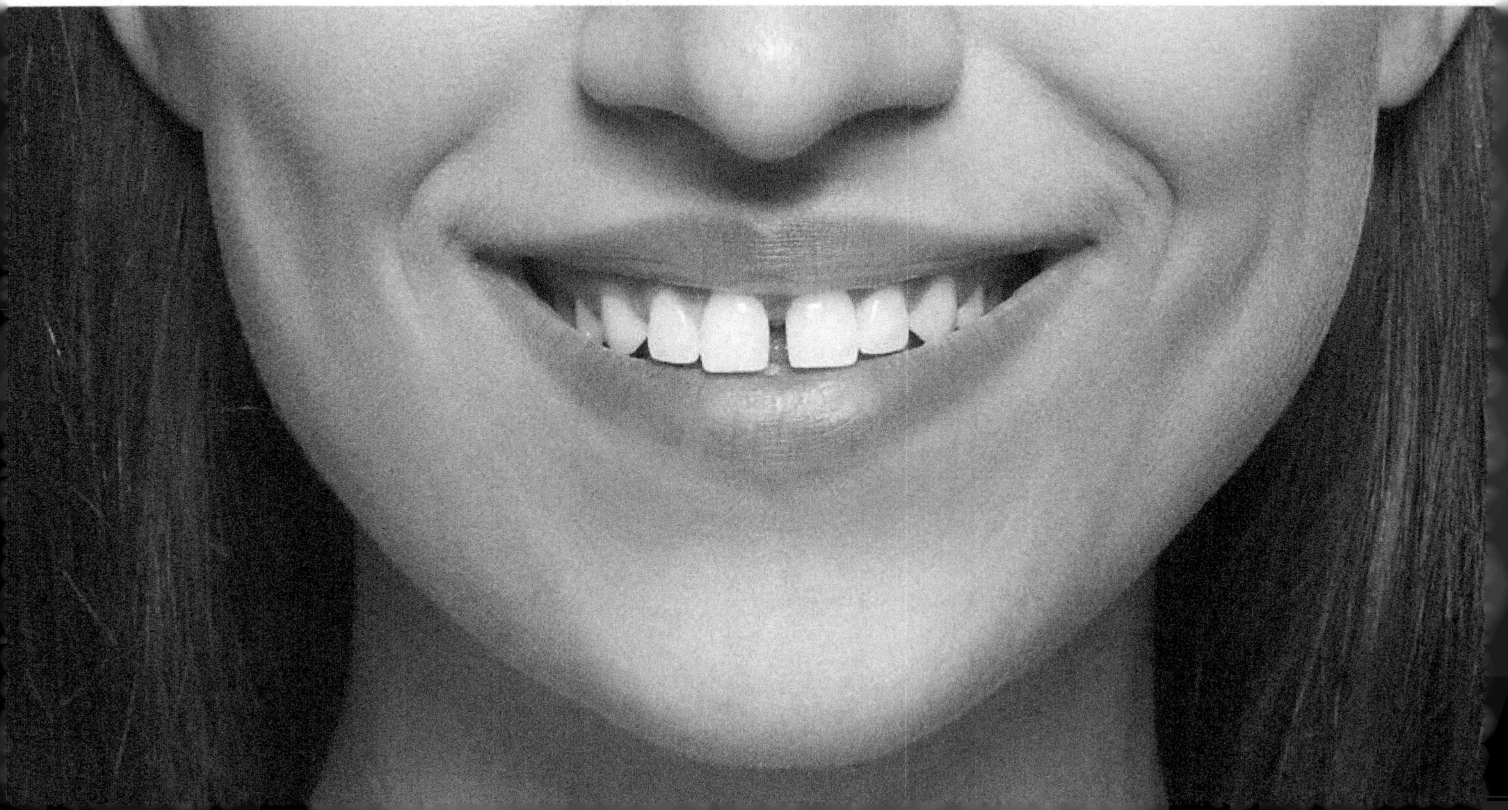

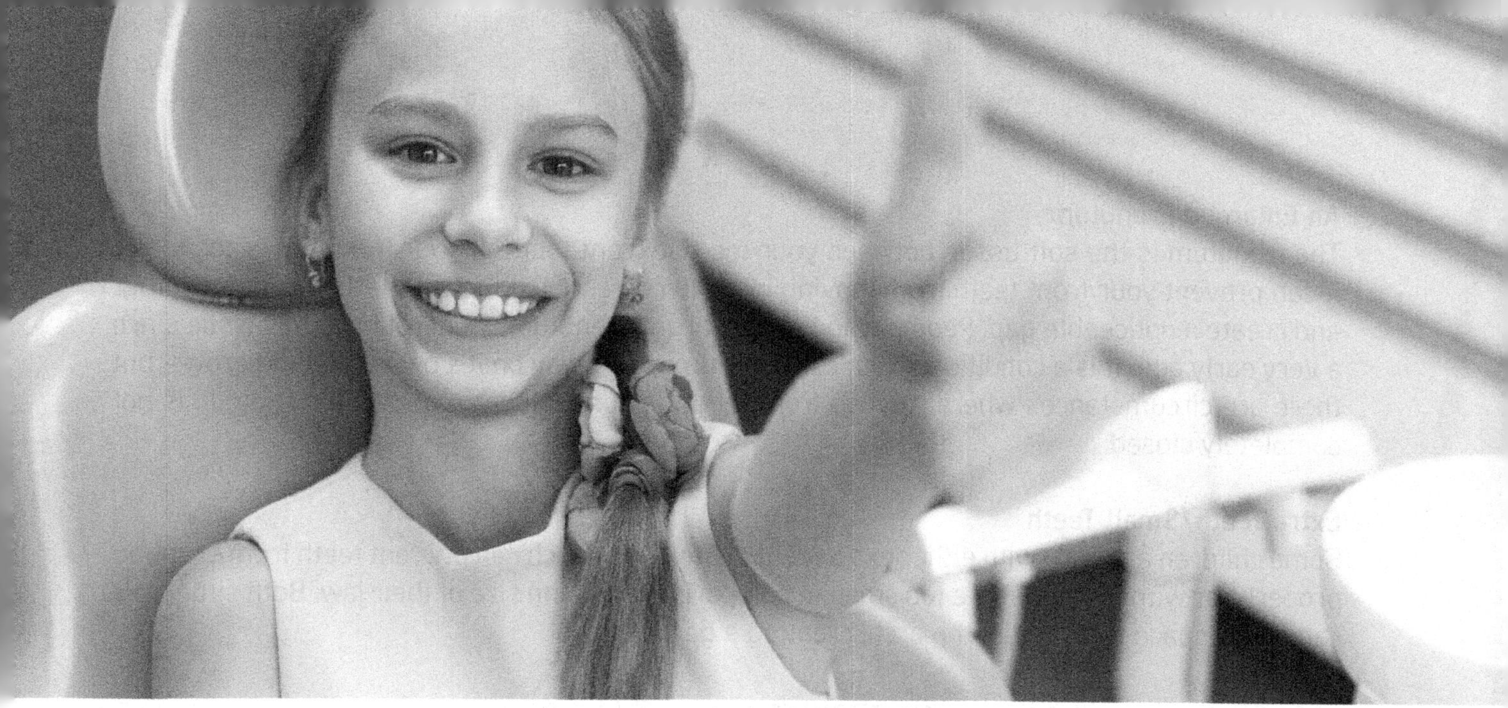

Some of the situations which can cause gap teeth include:

Use of a Pacifier/Thumbsucking
Both using a pacifier and thumbsucking are normal and soothing habits for babies and toddlers. They can be harmful, however, if the habits continue past the age where a child's permanent teeth have begun to erupt and position themselves into the mouth. This is because both habits push the tongue against the front teeth, causing them to be gradually moved out of their proper alignment. Over time, the space that is created may require dental care to fix so that other issues, such as a misalignment of the jaw, do not occur.

Tongue Thrusting
Tongue thrusting is a swallowing reflex that causes your tongue to push up against your top front teeth, causing gaps to develop over time.

Missing Teeth
If you are missing teeth or some of your adult teeth never erupted, the rest of your teeth can shift positions, causing gaps and other spacing problems.

An Enlarged Frenulum

The frenulum is the soft tissue between your top two front teeth. If your frenulum is too large, it can prevent your front teeth from moving into the correct position where they come together and create a noticeable gap. People who have enlarged frenulums general have this issue since a very early age. It is a condition which can sometimes go away on it's own as a child grows, but there are circumstances where the two front teeth do come closer together but the gap is not completely closed.

Extra Teeth/Small Teeth

Some children are born with either extra teeth in the bone which can prevent teeth from erupting properly, or with teeth that are too small in comparison with the size of their jaw. Both situations can cause space to be left in the arch, creating a gap.

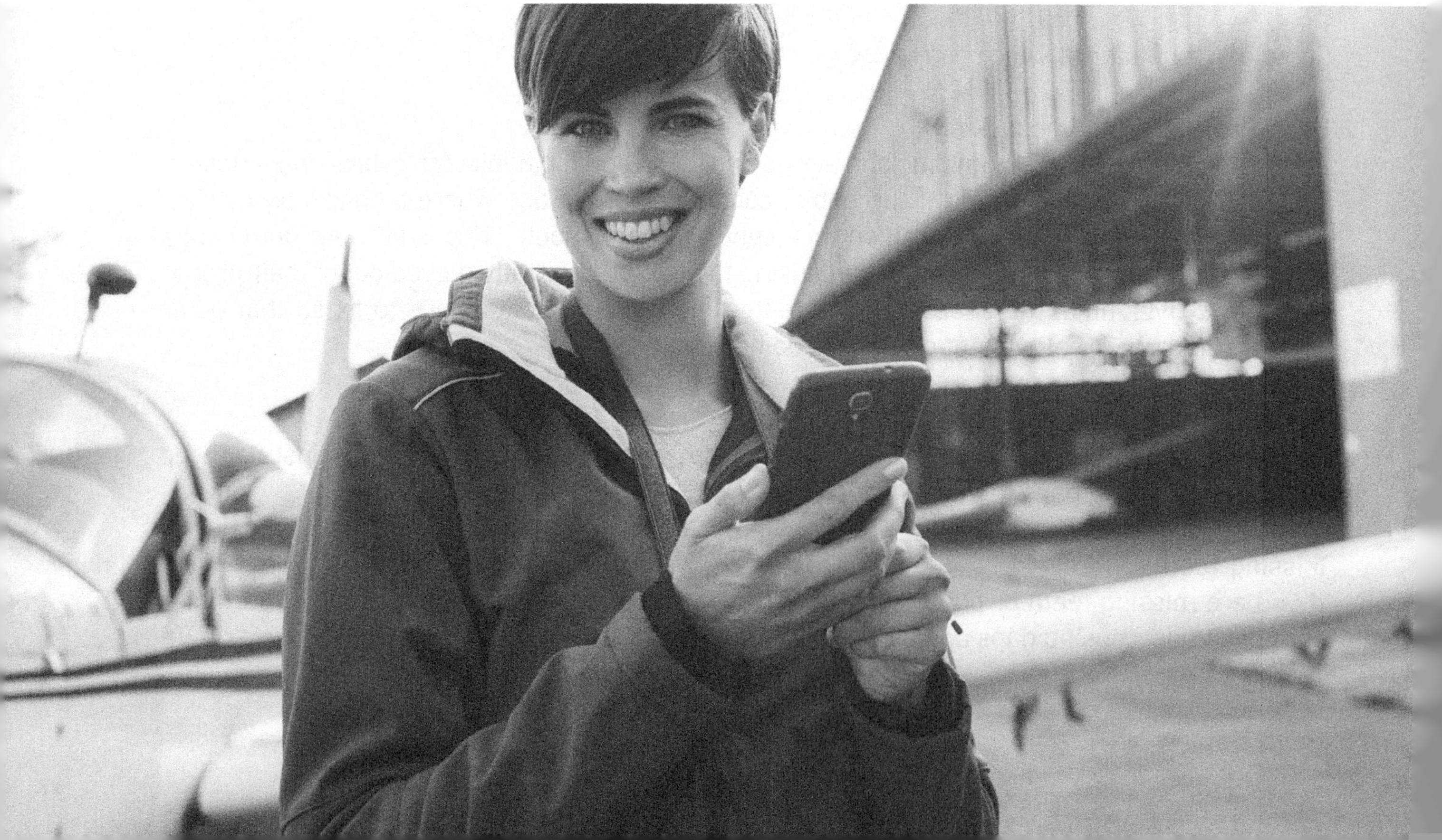

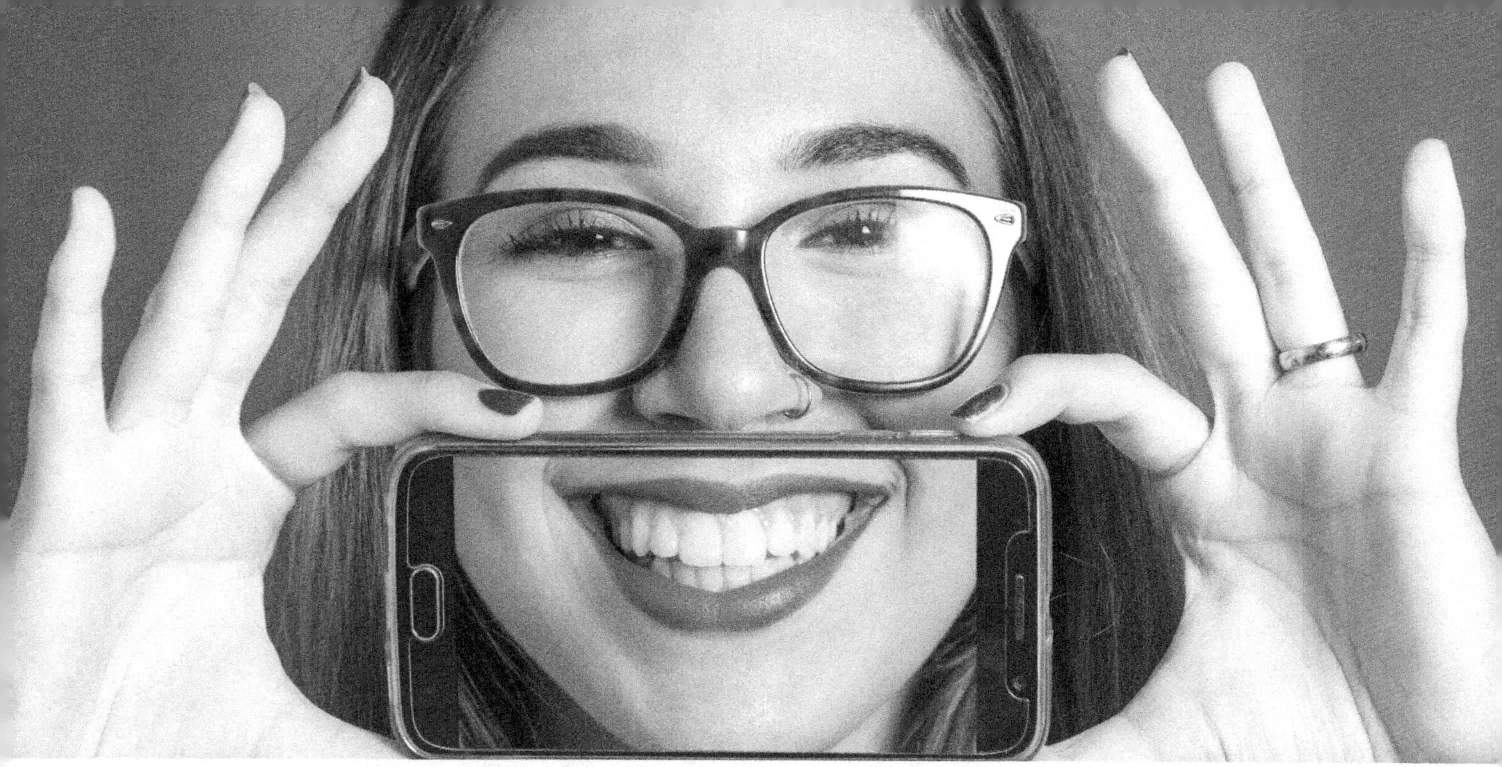

As discussed previously, the problem with gapped teeth is mostly one of aesthetics – many people are self-conscious about the gap and since it tends to be highly visible. However, there are some health issues which can occur from gap teeth where spacing issues can cause a problem with your bite later in life. Gap teeth also put you at an increased risk for gum disease and tooth decay, as having increased space between teeth can allow plaque to accumulate between them.

Invisalign is one of the best ways to treat gap teeth, as it offers a way to fix the problem without the added stigma of metal braces. It is also a pain free and works in a shorter amount of time than traditional braces.

TS Orthodontics is one of NC's top Invisalign providers. Please contact us at 828-254-4602 or visit our website at www.mytsosmile.com to set up your complimentary Smile Assessment.

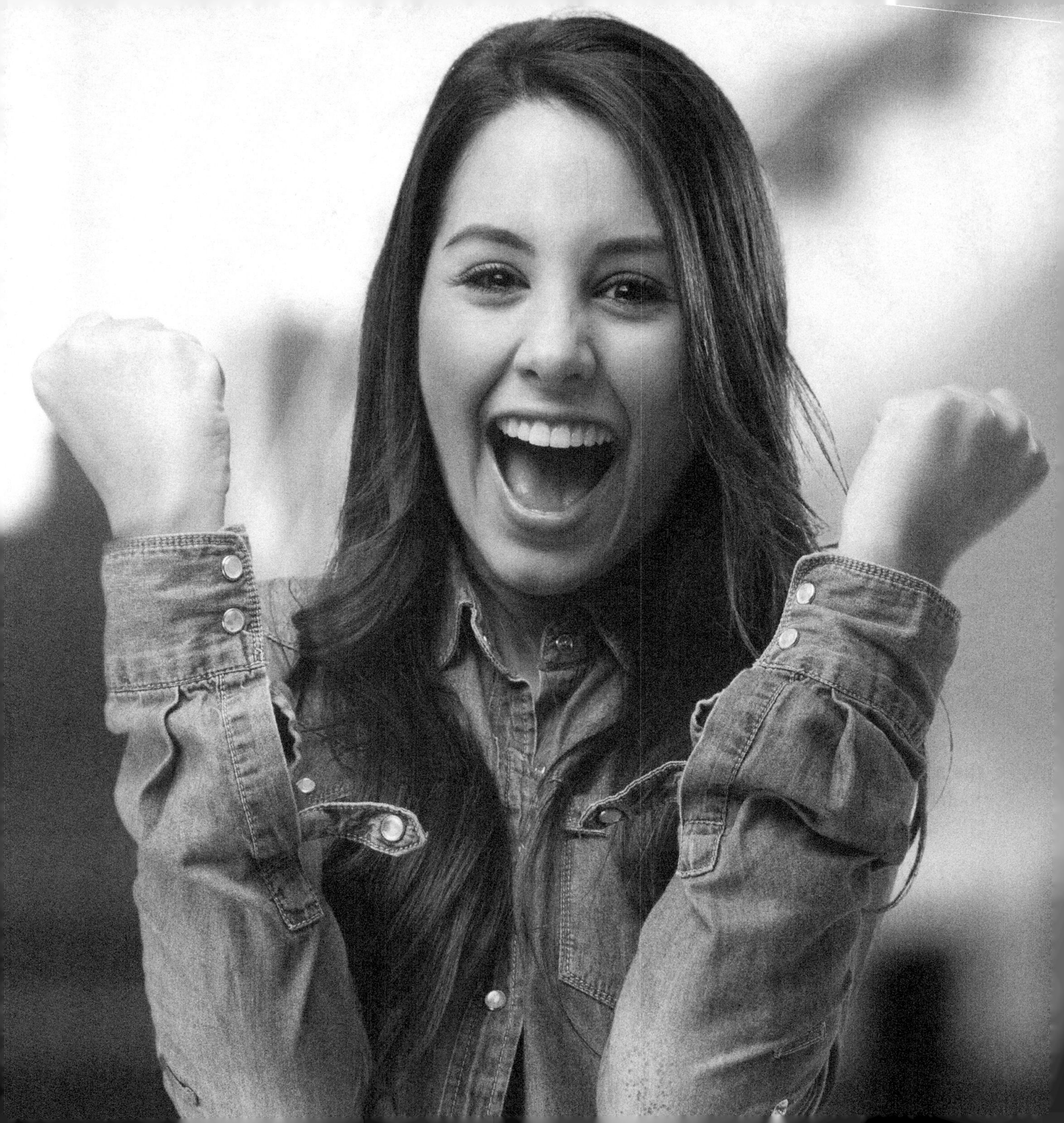

Open Bite

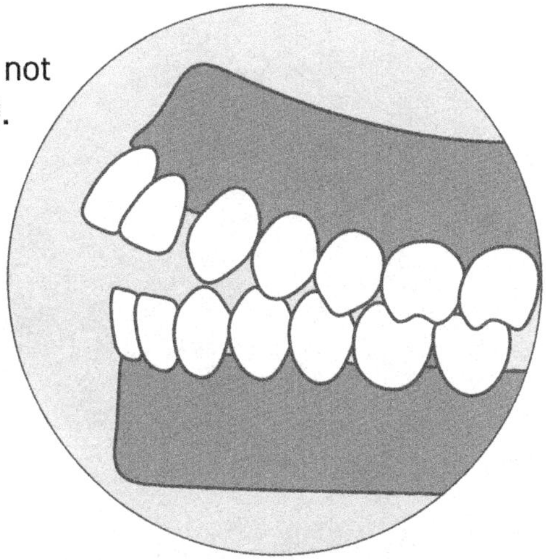

Open bite is a condition where your upper and lower teeth do not line up right, therefore they do not touch when your jaw is closed.

There are 3 major reasons why open bite occurs: skeletal, which is hereditary, dental, which occurs when baby teeth are mixed in with adult teeth, and due to a habit which has caused the jaw to shift, causing the misalignment and prohibiting closure.

Some of the habits which can cause open bite are:

- Consistent sucking of the lower lip
- Thumbsucking or pacifier use past the age of 2

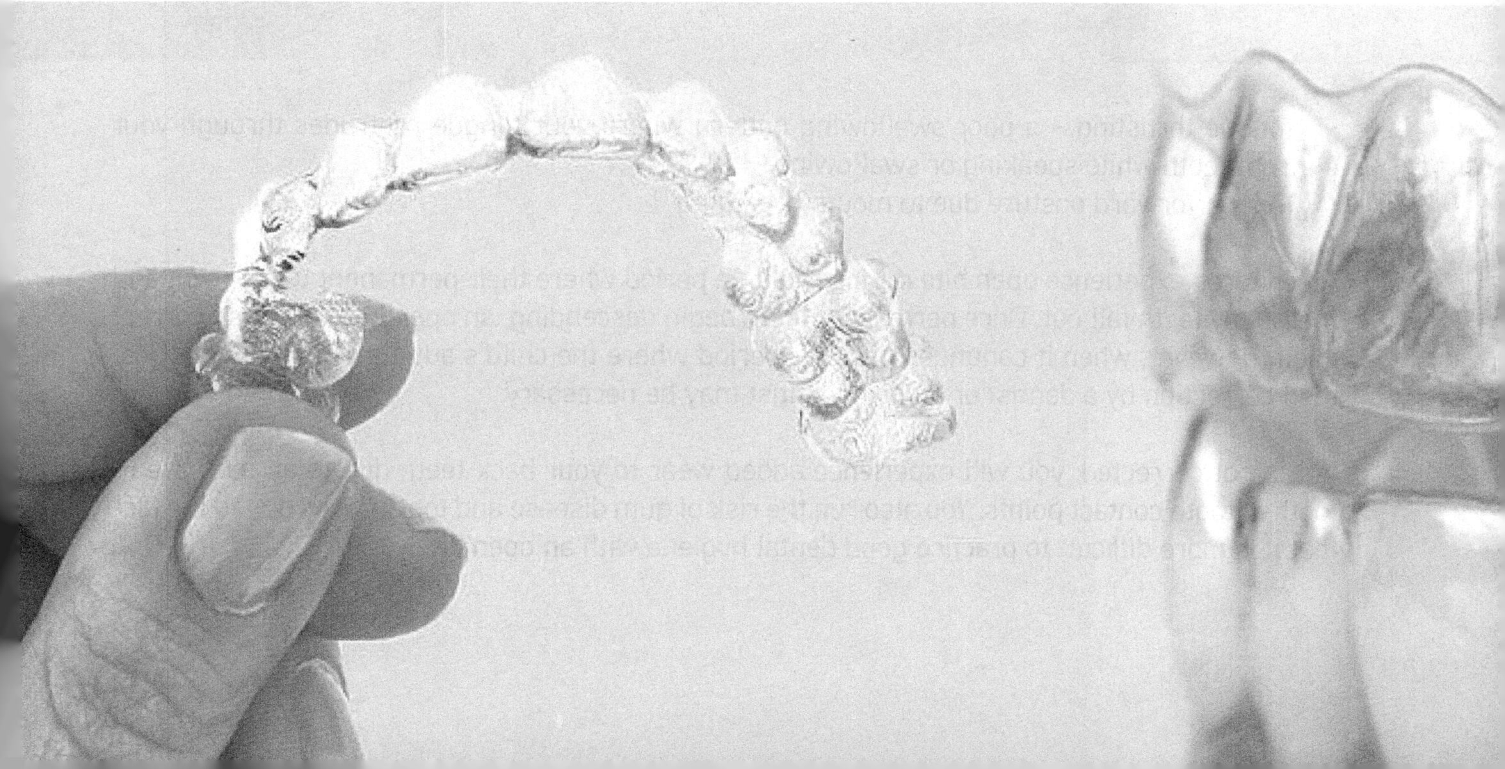

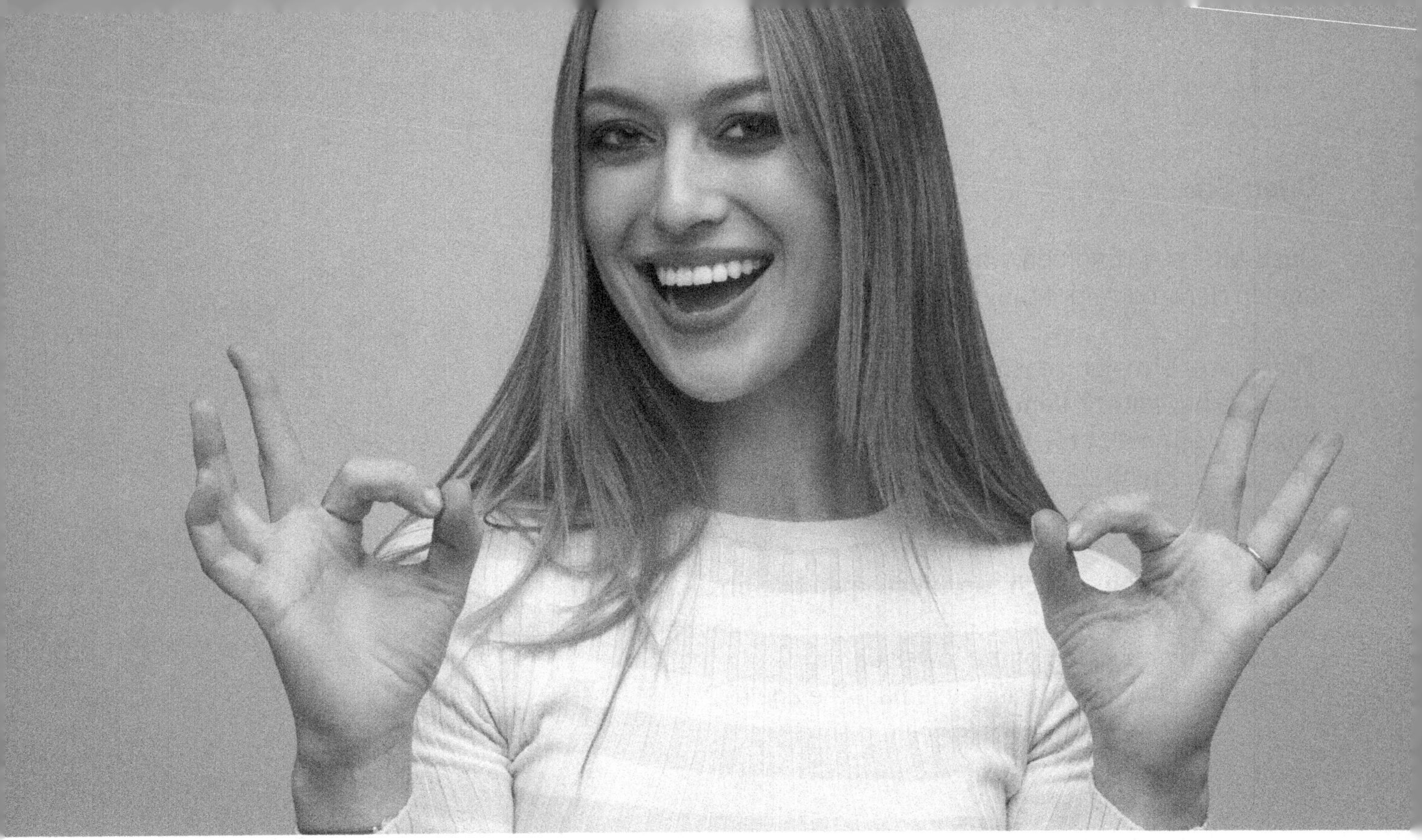

- Tongue thrusting – a poor swallowing pattern where your tongue protrudes through your front teeth while speaking or swallowing
- Tongue-forward posture due to mouth breathing

All children experience open bite during the time period where their permanent teeth erupt and their baby teeth fall out. Once permanent teeth begin descending, an open bite will often correct itself. However, when it continues past the period where the child's adult teeth have emerged, then correction by a dentist or an orthodontist may be necessary.

If it is not corrected, you will experience added wear to your back teeth due to an increase in tooth to tooth contact points. You also run the risk of gum disease and tooth decay due to the fact that it is more difficult to practice good dental hygiene with an open bite.

Biting into foods such as apples can very difficult with an open bite. Chewing is also very painful. Many children with this condition work around pain while chewing by not properly breaking their food down before swallowing. This can create serious digestive issues in future in addition to jaw pain.

Speech impairment can occur in children who do not have their open bite treated.

One additional concern of not treating an open bite is that this condition makes it difficult – and in some severe cases, impossible – to prevent food or liquids from escaping the mouth while eating and drinking unless you put your tongue in the gap to stop it. This can create an awkward and uncomfortable social situation for the child, and it can cause embarrassment or the urge to withdraw from eating around others.

In the past, open bite required metal braces and in more severe cases, surgery to correct. Today, Invisalign is an effective method of treating many open bite cases by pushing your teeth into the proper position gradually. This method is less painful and requires less time for correction, and you get all of the benefits of Invisalign over traditional braces included!

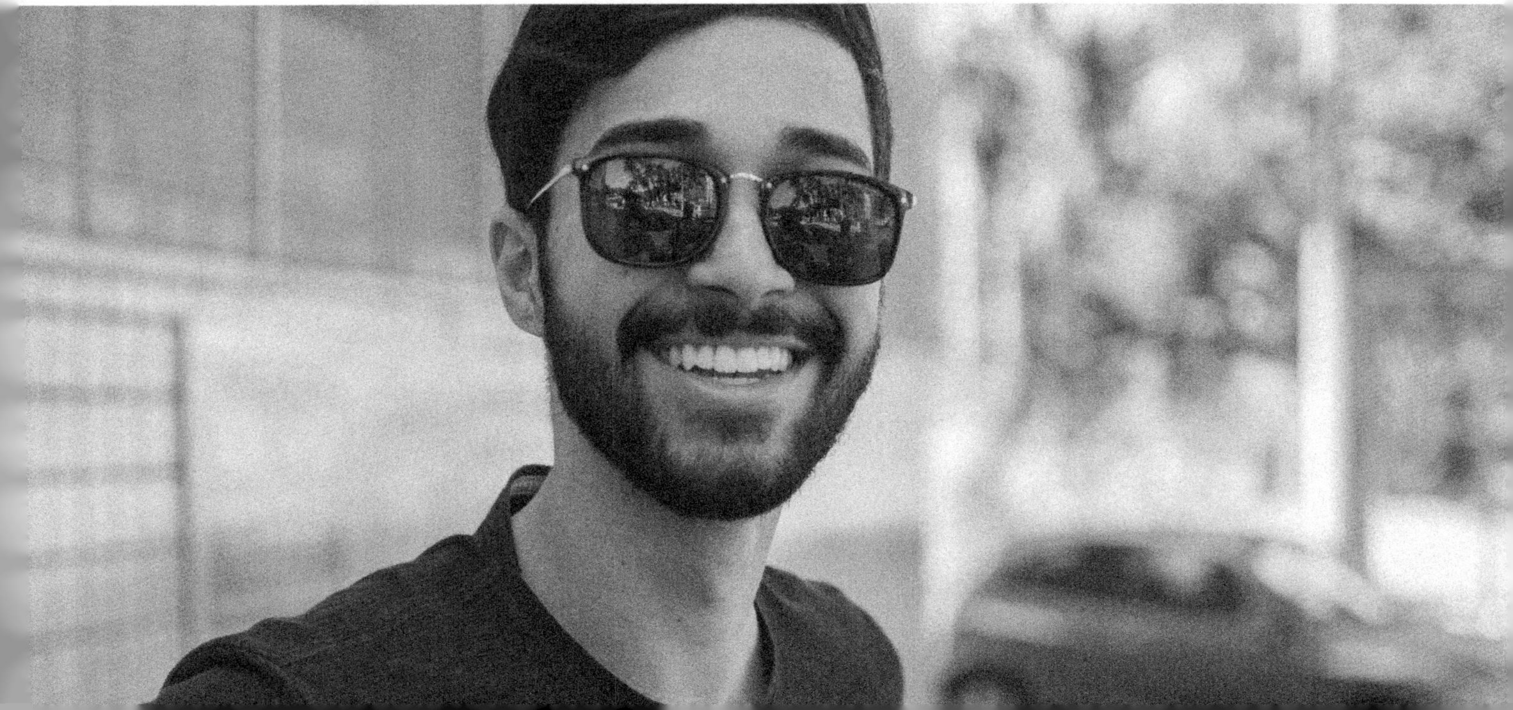

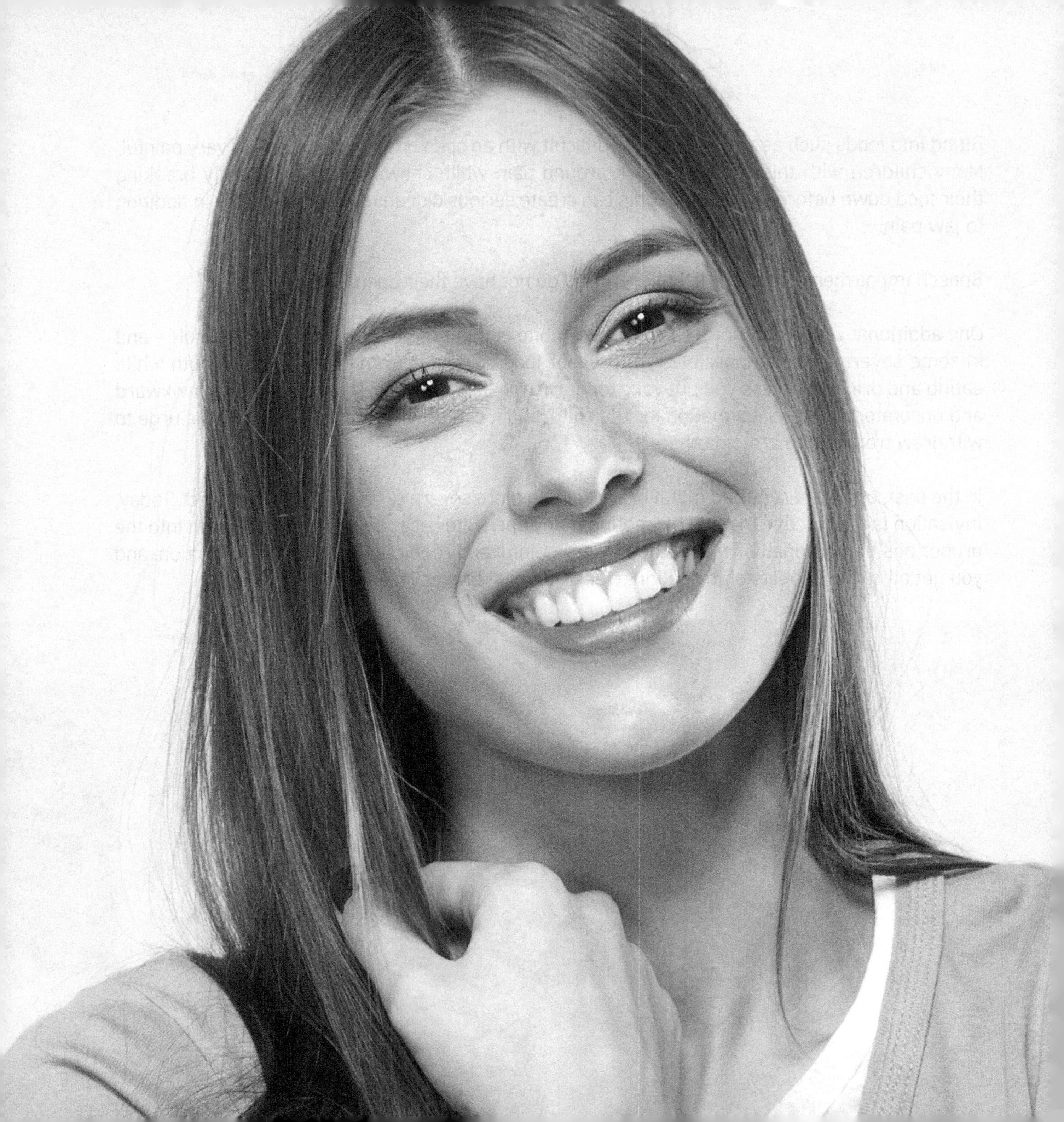

General Teeth Straightening

The aim of this book is to help you make an informed decision about Invisalign and whether or not it is the right choice for you or your teen. There are a number of smile abnormalities that Invisalign can correct, and the benefit of doing so in less time and with minimal interruption to your daily life is undoubtedly one of the biggest reasons why we recommend it to the patients in our practice.

But...what if you do not have a condition that requires major orthodontic correction? What if you just want to have straighter teeth?

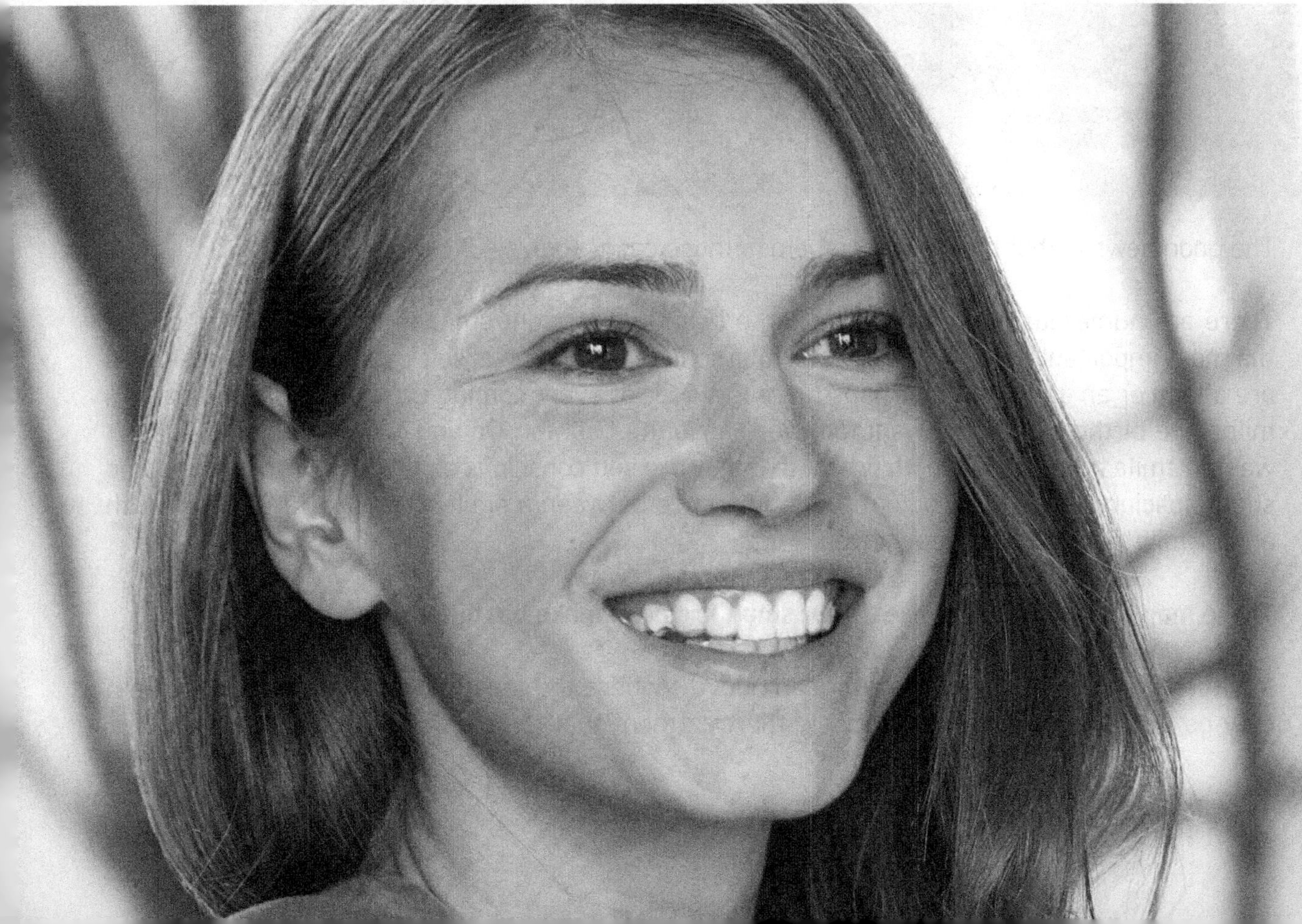

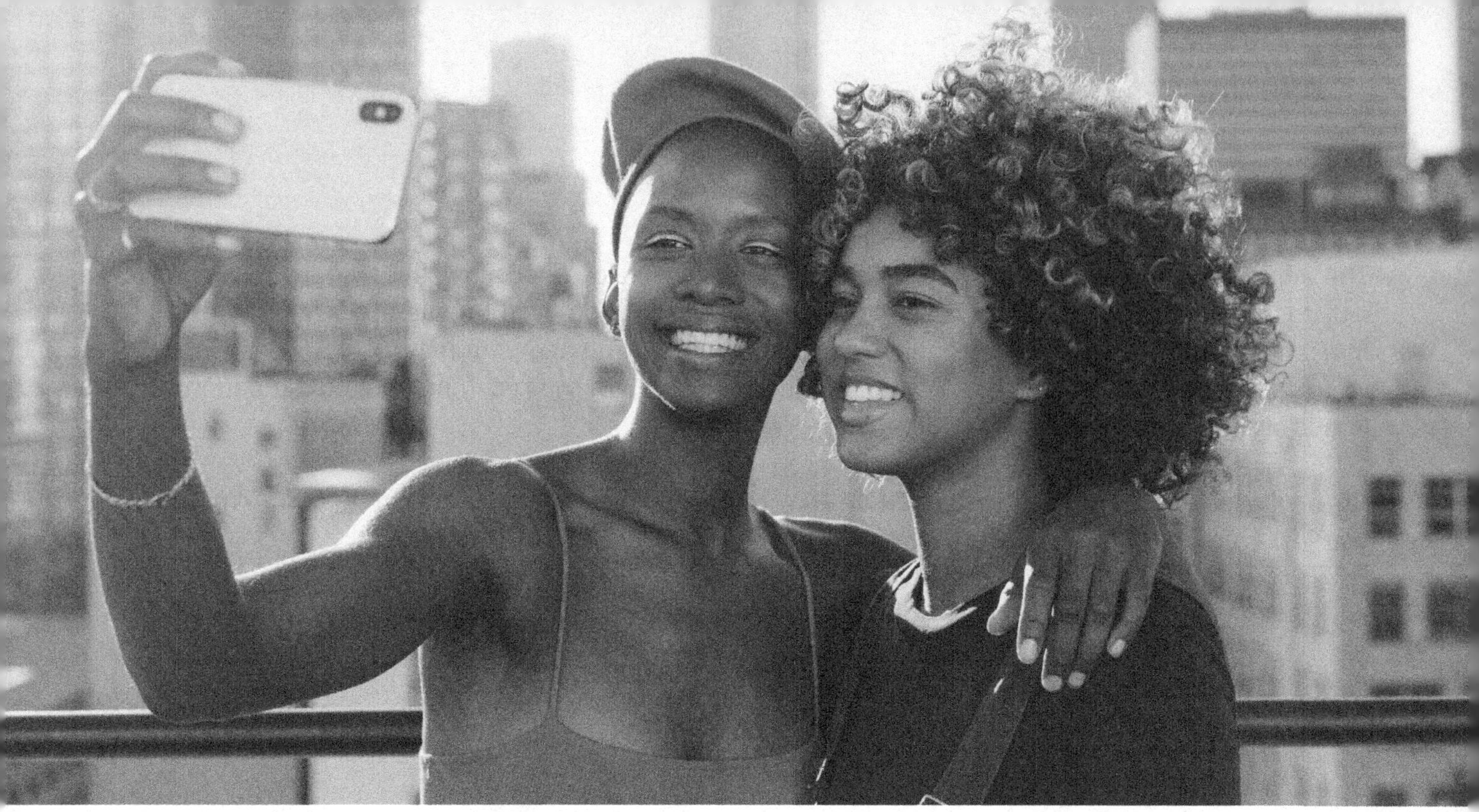

The good news is that Invisalign can help in those cases too!

There are numerous reasons why having a beautiful, straight smile is important, with one of the most important being that it boosts your confidence and your self-esteem regardless if you are a teen or an adult. But...perhaps there is a special event coming up such as a wedding or a milestone birthday that you want look your absolute best for. Or, you have a teen that doesn't want to smile because of a tooth or two that they are self conscious about. Maybe you have some slight spacing issues that could make a difference between a smile that you are "just ok" with and a smile that you absolutely love.

These may sound like small fixes – but small fixes can make big differences.

In situations such as the ones described above - where the a patient's issues with their teeth may be minor – Invisalign is precisely the treatment that is best suited to make corrections.

Because it is not intrusive, virtually unnoticeable, and takes far less time than traditional braces, it is an excellent choice for improving your appearance and your overall, long term health – regardless of age.
And let's face it - smiling makes you not just look good, but feel good too. In fact, this is something that has been proven by countless studies by both scientist and health professionals!

The act of smiling activates the neural messaging in your brain. It releases a substance called neuropeptides. These tiny molecules allow neurons to communicate - in other words, they are the messenger for your emotions. When you feel sad, happy, angry, stressed or excited - they spring into action by fighting of stress. When you smile, you activate the "feel good" transmitters that your body naturally has: endorphins, seratonin, and dopamine. All of this together relaxes you body, lowers your heart rate, and levels your blood pressure.

Endorphins also act as a pain reliever - one that is one hundred percent healthy and organic. Releasing them naturally makes your body feel better. Serotonin has similar effects by acting as a mood lifter and natural antidepressant.

Since there are so many reasons to smile - including some which are proven to be good for your overall health and wellbeing...you should try to do it as much as possible. And with Invisalign, you can do so with confidence and with a beautiful, healthy smile that will make others around you want to smile too!

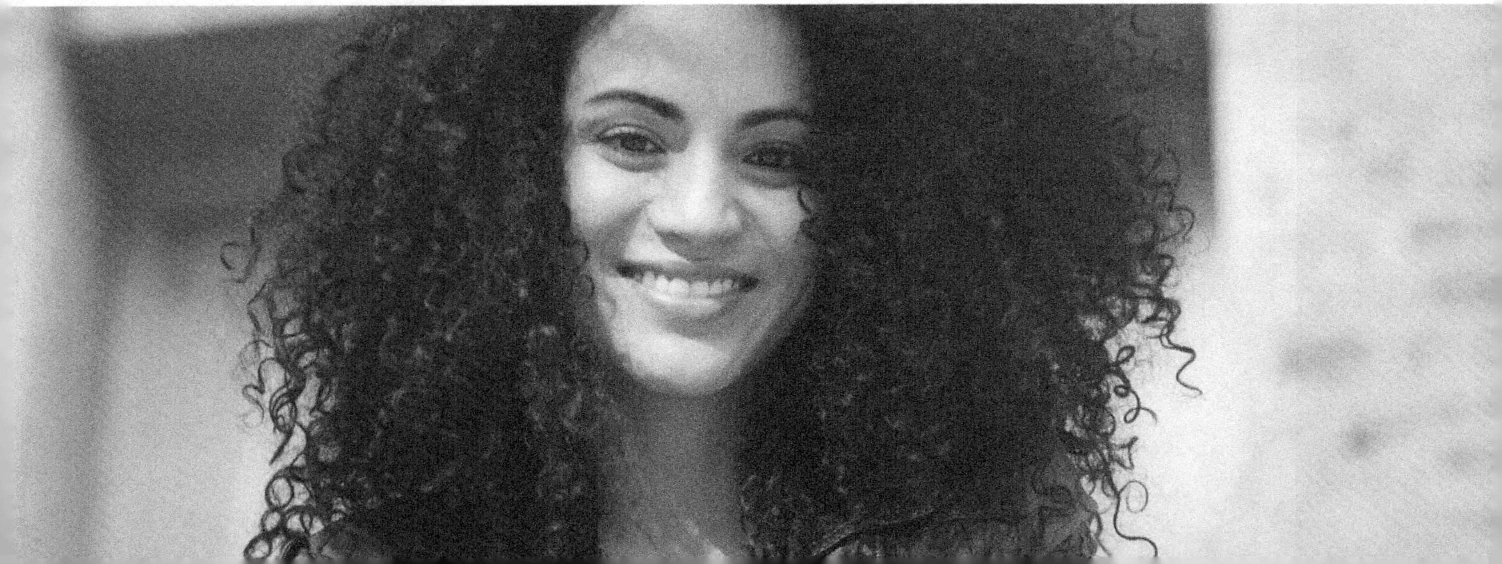

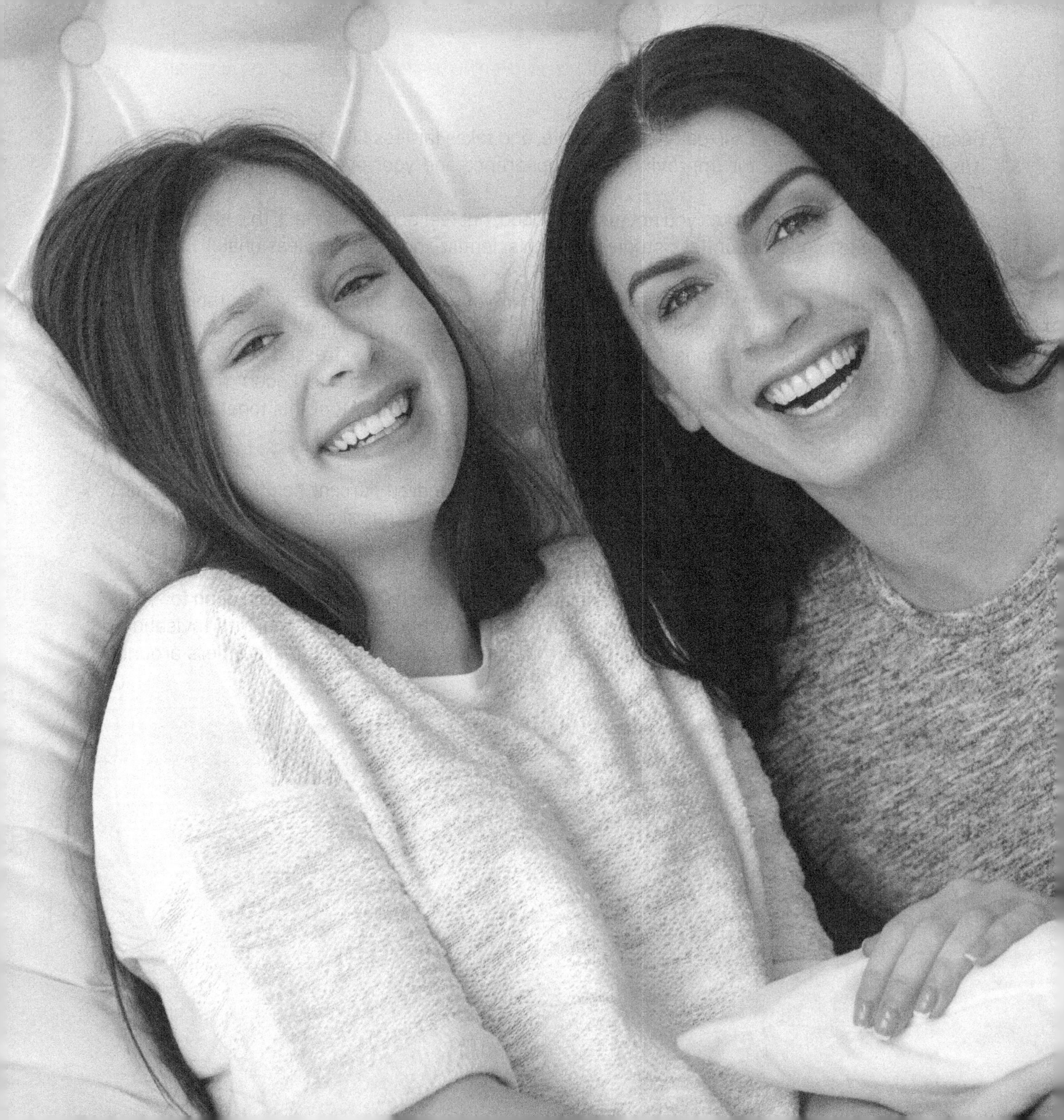

Chapter 5: The Cost of Invisalign

One of the biggest questions that patients ask about Invisalign is whether or not it is more expensive than traditional metal braces. And the answer is...it depends! While in the past, Invisalign was a bit more cost prohibitive, today it is a common treatment and it is comparatively priced to traditional braces. It must be assessed on a case-by-case basis as no patients - or their teeth - are exactly the same.

Some of the main factors that determine Invisalign's cost is how long you will need to be in treatment and what type of dental issues need to be fixed.

The best way to calculate what your overall cost will be is by scheduling a consultation with an orthodontist. During your consultation, which most orthodontists offer at no cost, you can determine what your goals are for your smile, what your issues are that you wish or correct, and how you want to proceed with your treatment if you are a good candidate. You can also discuss any underlying health issues or concerns that you may have at that time.

TS Orthodontics is one of NC's top Invisalign providers. Please contact us at 828-254-4602 or visit our website at www.mytsosmile.com to set up your complimentary Smile Assessment.

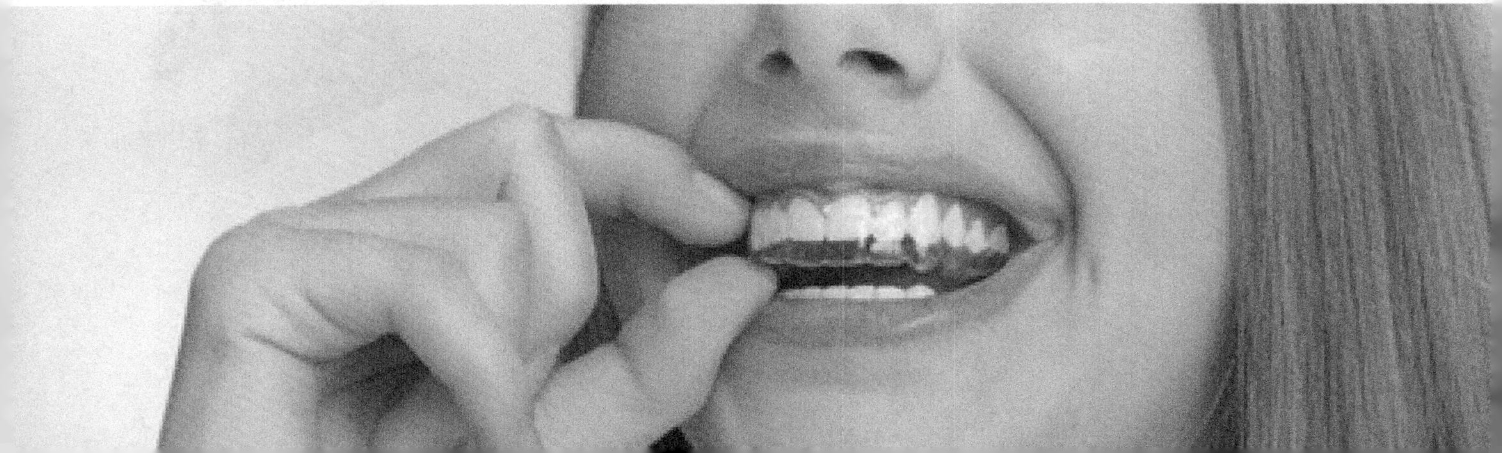

Another important factor to consider in price is patient cooperation and compliance. Patients who fail to wear their aligners as directed, miss appointments, or who practice poor oral hygiene run the risk of extending their treatment. If you do not take proper care of your trays, you may be hindered from moving on to the next step.

On the flip side of this - the more closely a patient follows the plan for treatment outlined by their doctor, the less time it will take to complete it.

How long you are in treatment directly affects the cost of treatment. Therefore it should be your goal to follow your doctor's guidelines for compliance so that you can get your treatment completed in a time frame that works for you - and at a cost that works for you too!

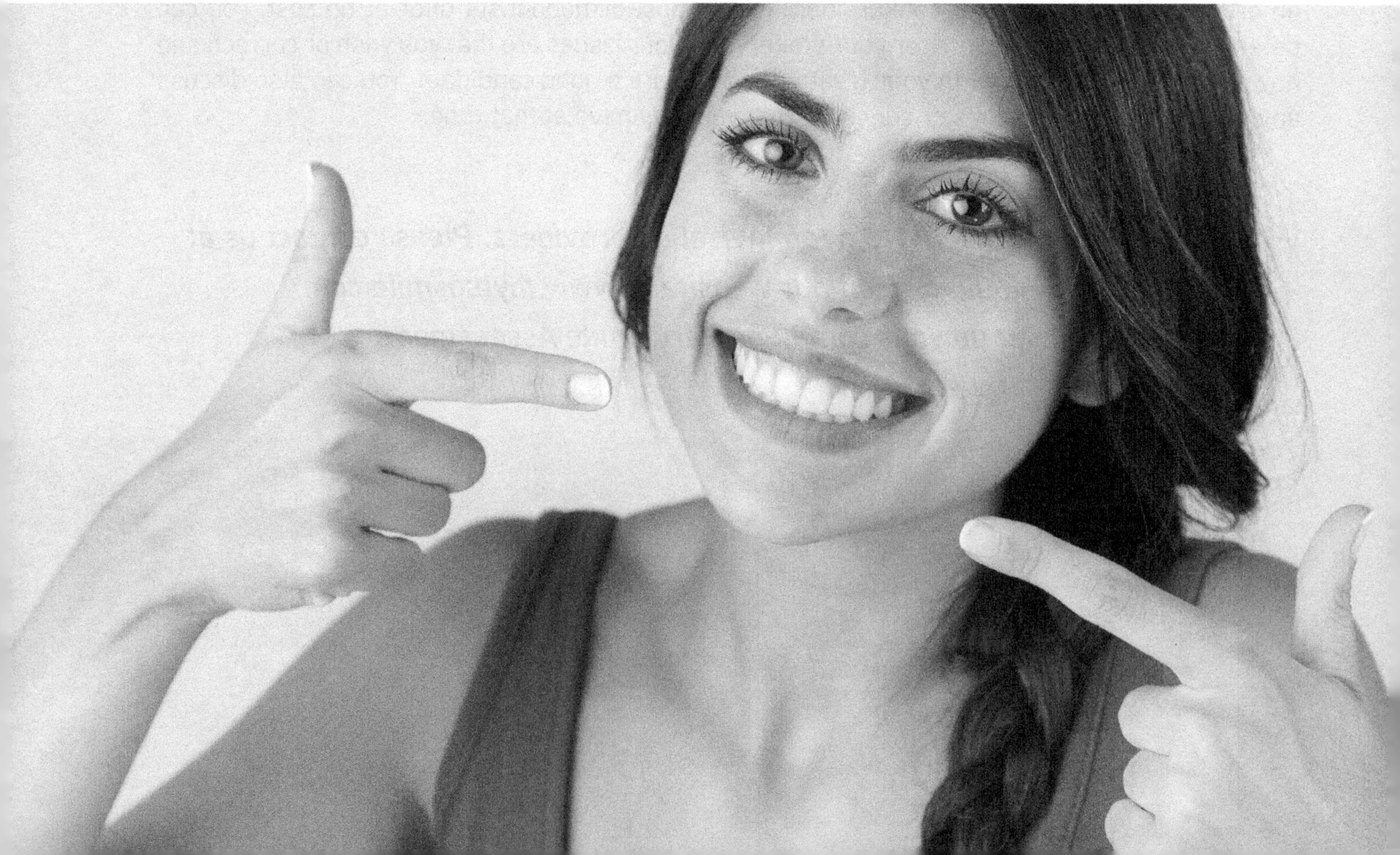

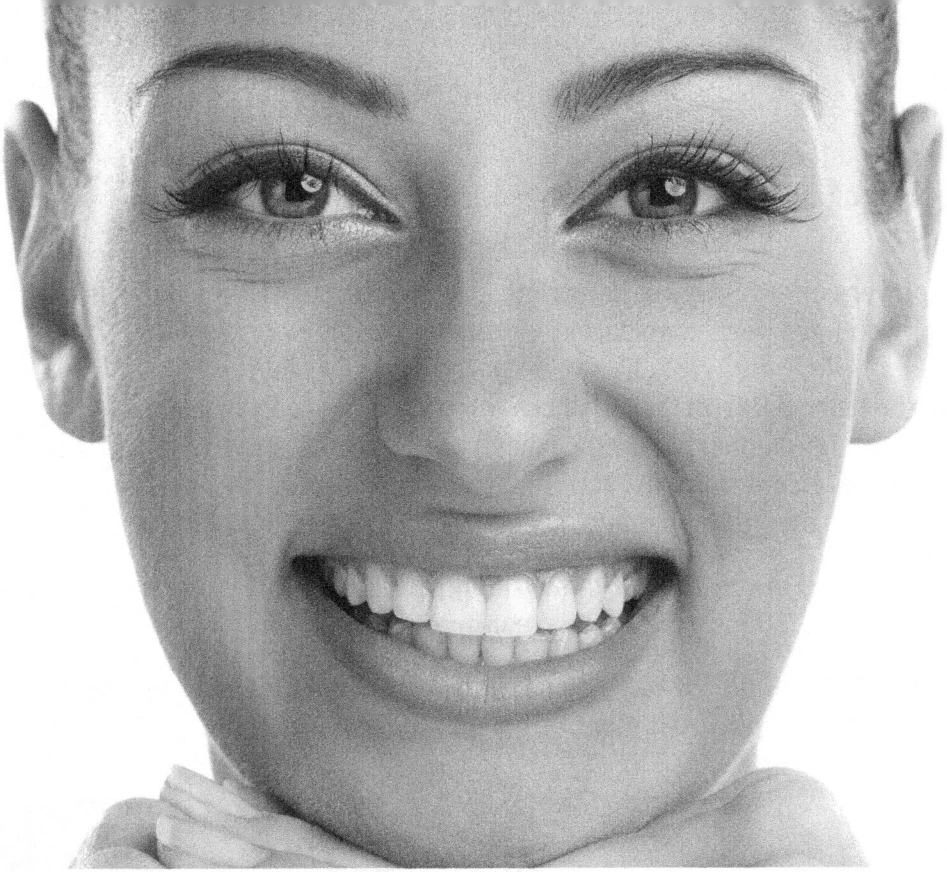

Ways to Pay for Invisalign Treatment

Here are a few ways you can pay for Invisalign which will help make it more attainable for you or your family.

- **Use your Flexible Savings Account (FSA).** Through some employers, patients can take advantage of creating an FSA. This allows patients to set aside a set amount of money from their paycheck to be used on medical, dental and orthodontic costs, including Invisalign aligners.

  Your FSA is managed by your employer and the current federal guidelines at the time of this writing allow for you to set aside up to $2,600 per year in this account.

A large benefit of an FSA is that you do not pay taxes on any money that you put into this account.

Not all employers offer FSAs, but be sure to check with yours to see if this is offered at your workplace if you have been considering Invisalign.

- **Consider getting a Health Savings Account (HSA).** This account is designed for individuals who have a high-deductible on their health insurance plan. It works similarly to an FSA in that you put money into this account in incremental deposits and this money is utilized specifically for medical and dental costs, including Invisalign aligners.

  Current laws as of the time of this writing permit you to set aside up to $3,400 for an individual or $6,750 for a family per year in an HSA.

Much like an FSA, you do not pay taxes on any money you allocate to this account, but in order to open an HSA, you must meet IRS eligibility requirements.

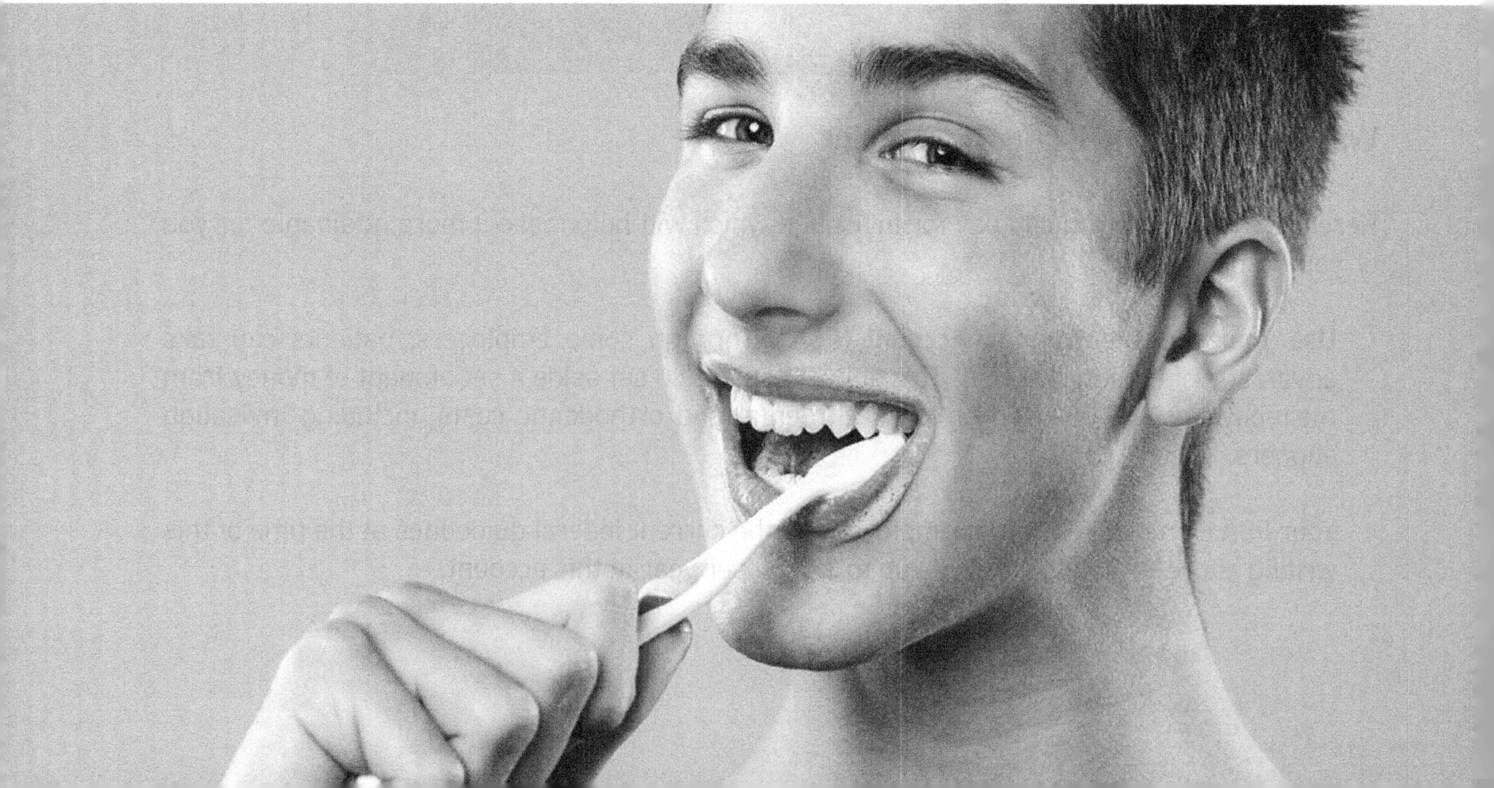

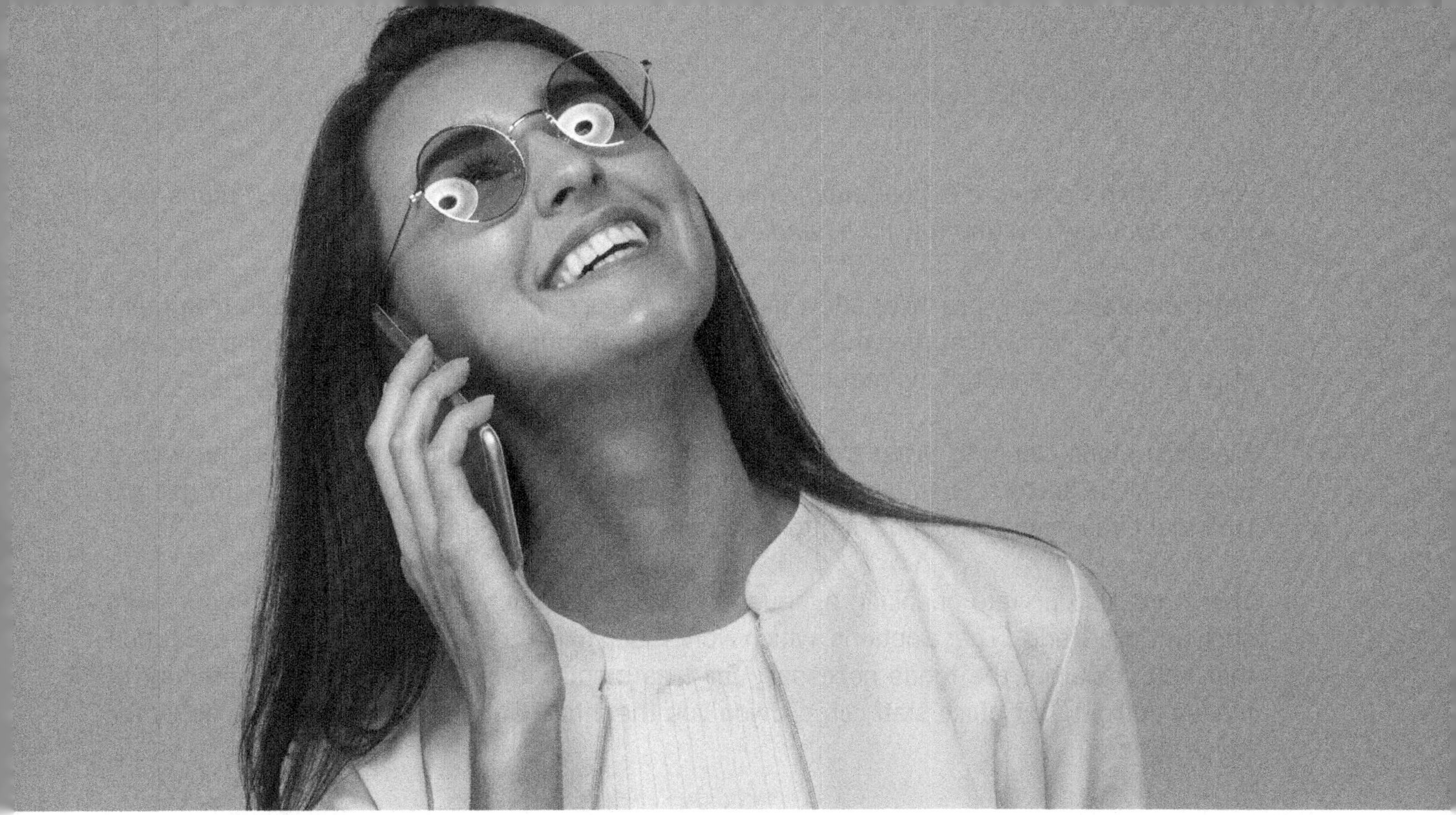

Note: before beginning your treatment, talk to your doctor's office and your benefits manager to determine if your provider can pay the doctor directly for your treatment, or if you will need to pay for treatment and be reimbursed from your FSA or HSA.

- **Dental insurance.** Many dental insurance plans cover Invisalign aligners in the same way that they cover braces. How much of the cost of your treatment will be paid by insurance and how much will be out of pocket depends on your plan.

  Some insurance providers, however, consider orthodontic treatment to be an elective service and therefore do not cover it. In many cases, the providers that do cover it frequently have a lifetime cap on how much care they will pay for. Therefore, be sure to check with your benefits manager or your insurance company's customer service center on what your plan's particulars are in this area.

Note: When booking a consultation, check with the doctor's office to see which plans they accept and how treatment will be handled from a payment standpoint.

- **Payment plans.** Many practices allow patients to make monthly payments for their treatment through a plan that will spread the cost of Invisalign throughout the length of your treatment. Most of these payment plans require a down payment before you can begin treatment.

  Payment plans can help bring treatment within reach to patients who are working with a budget. Most doctors offer plans that are flexible and affordable so that you can get the treatment you need without having to worry about how you will be able to pay for it.

  There are also private financing avenues available on which you can obtain on your own, such as CareCredit®. These options, which work much like a credit card does, can be a solution that helps you get the funds necessary for treatment without needing a large amount of money upfront. Our office staff can provide you the information needed on how to apply for these options.

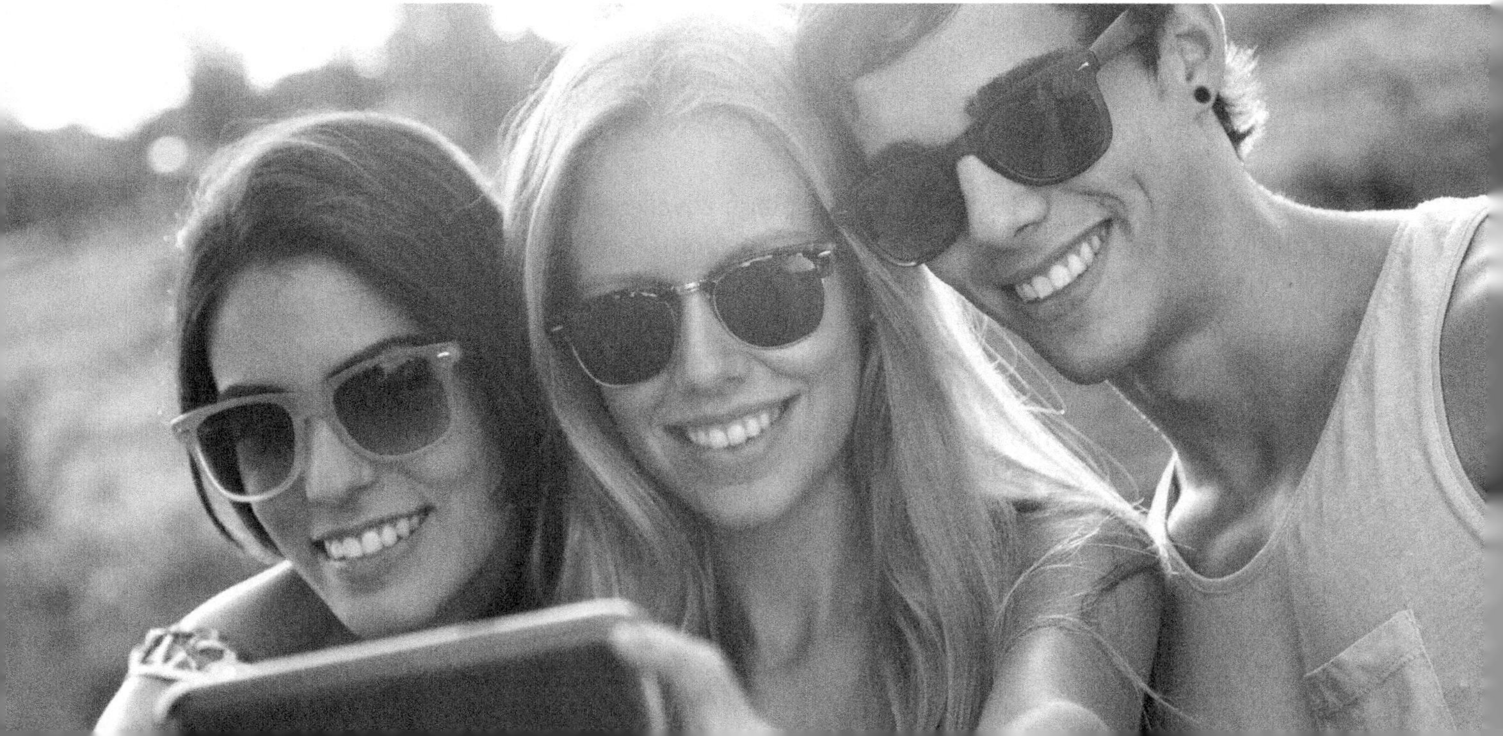

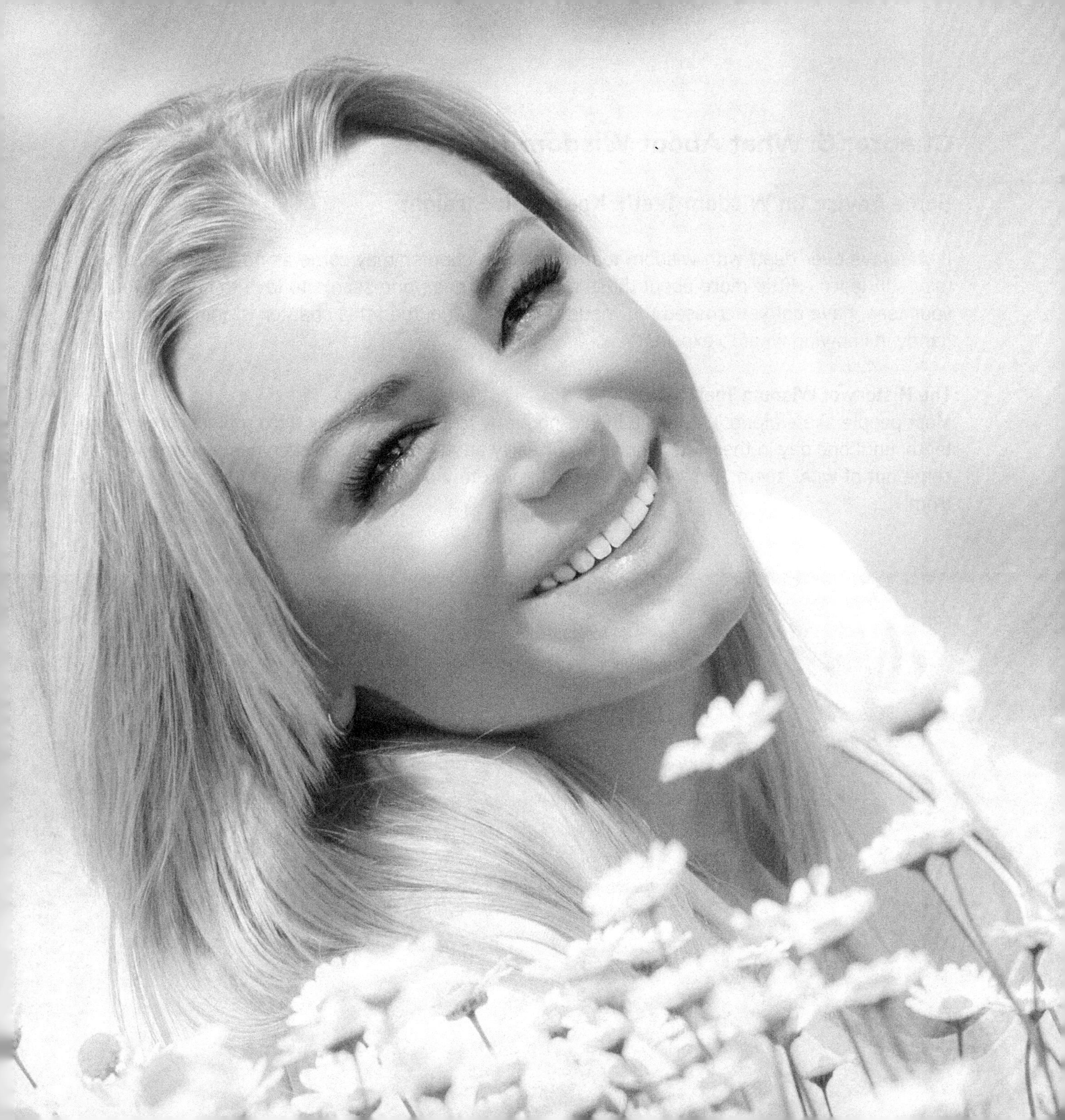

Chapter 6: What About Wisdom Teeth?

Some Advice On Wisdom Teeth: Keeping It Straight

If you have ever dealt with wisdom teeth, then this chapter may come as no surprise, yet you may still learn a little more about those molars that everyone seems to love to hate. If you, or your teen, have not yet crossed the wisdom teeth bridge, then this chapter is going to come in handy in knowing what to expect.

The History of Wisdom Teeth

Most people skate along just fine in life without any trouble from their third molars, or wisdom teeth, until one day in their late teen years or early adulthood, when it becomes an issue. It may come out of what seems like nowhere, leaving you to wonder exactly where those teeth came from!

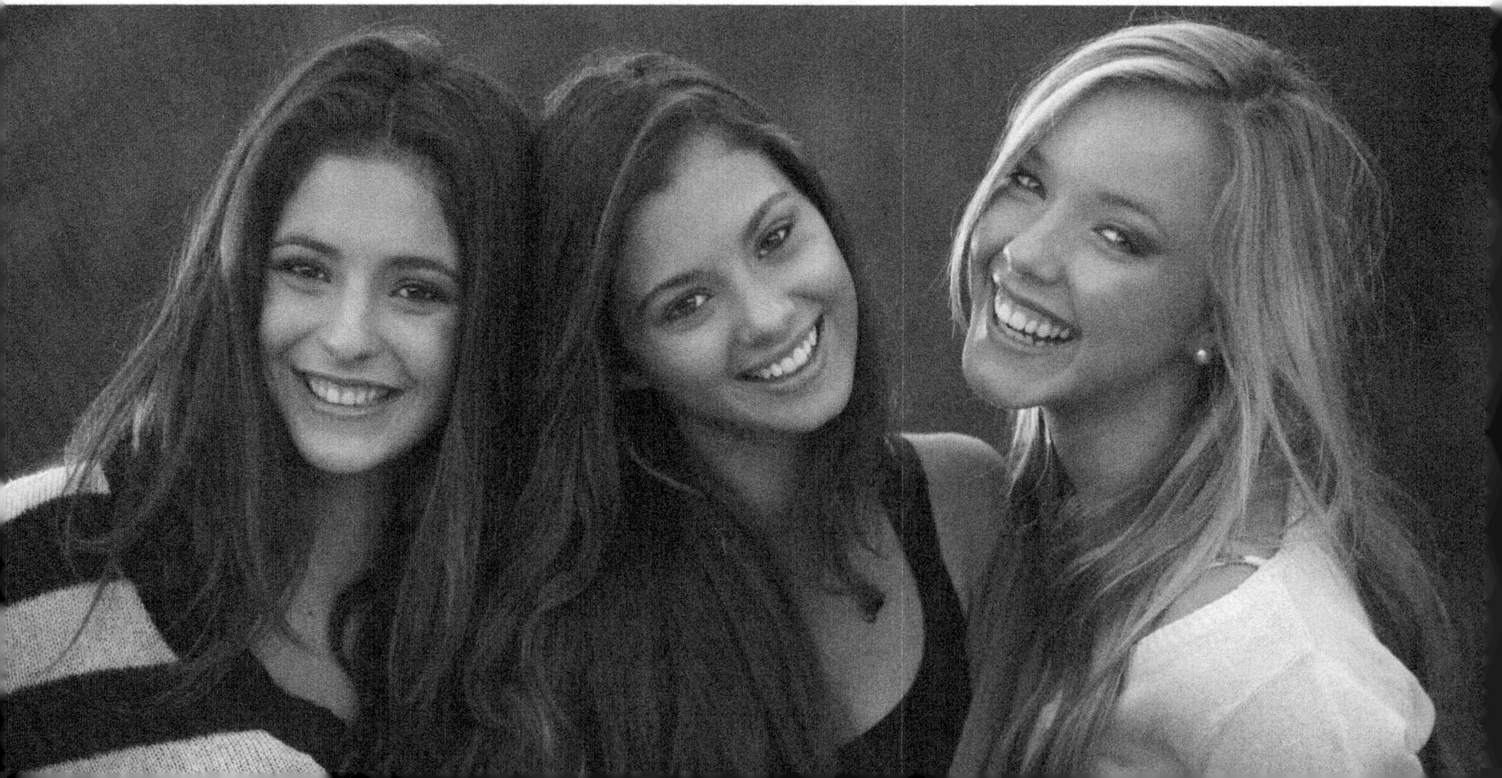

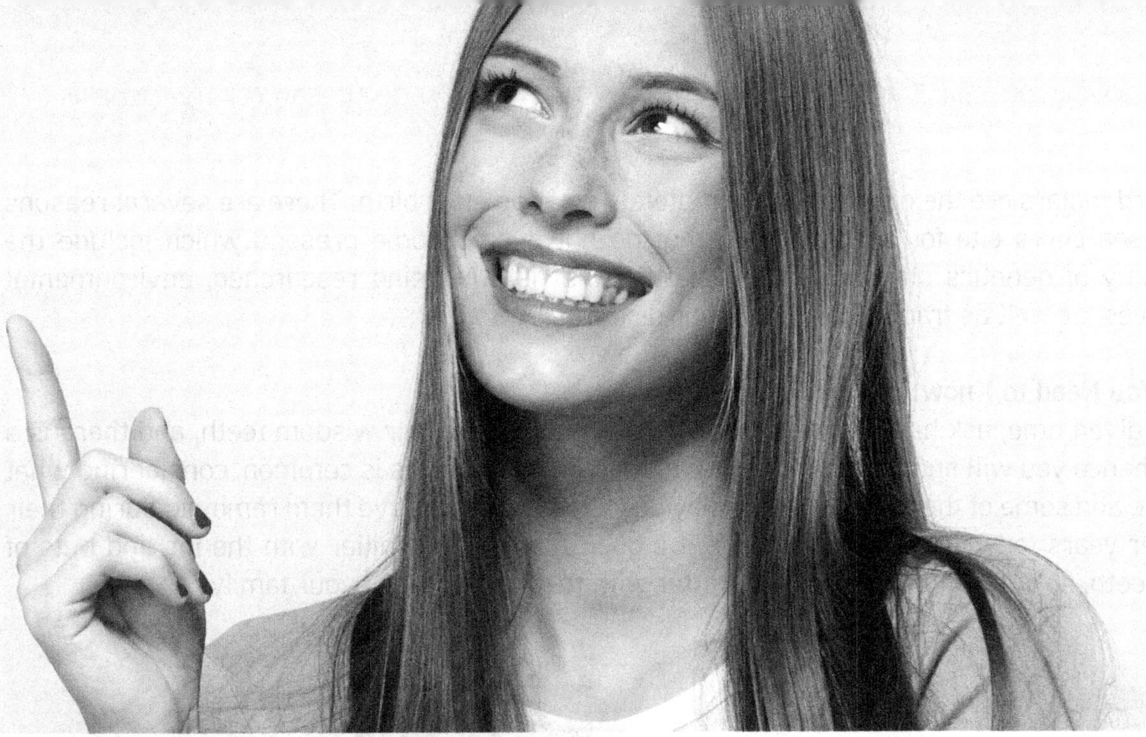

It's a good question, too. While it seems like the wisdom teeth come from out of nowhere and just start posing a problem one day, they actually have a long established history and began making their way long before you ever noticed them. Scientists believe that the wisdom teeth once served an important purpose thousands of years ago.

Our ancestors ate a lot of food that was tougher and chewier, such as leaves, roots, and even some raw meat. It's believed that this diet was harsher on the teeth, causing them to wear down faster., Because of this, we had a third set of molars, known as the wisdom teeth today, that would erupt to help carry the burden of all that chewing.

As things changed over time, including much of our diet and the shape of our jaw, our wisdom teeth have come to pose more of a problem for most people, rather than be an asset due to the fact that they now have a difficult time fitting into our jaw. Yet not everyone even has wisdom teeth that emerge. Around 35 percent of the population never have wisdom teeth that develop, something that makes a lot of other people envious of them!

The third molars are the only teeth to completely develop after birth. There are several reasons that researchers cite for wisdom teeth that do not ever become present, which include the possibility of genetics playing a role, although that is still being researched, environmental influences, as well as trauma to the head or diseases.

What You Need to Know About Wisdom Teeth

At any given time, ask half a dozen adults around you about their wisdom teeth, and there is a good chance you will find that most have had them removed. This is common, considering what they are and some of the risks that they may pose. Many people have them removed during their younger years for valid reasons, making it a good idea to be familiar with the ins and outs of these teeth, so you will be able to deal better with them for you and your family.

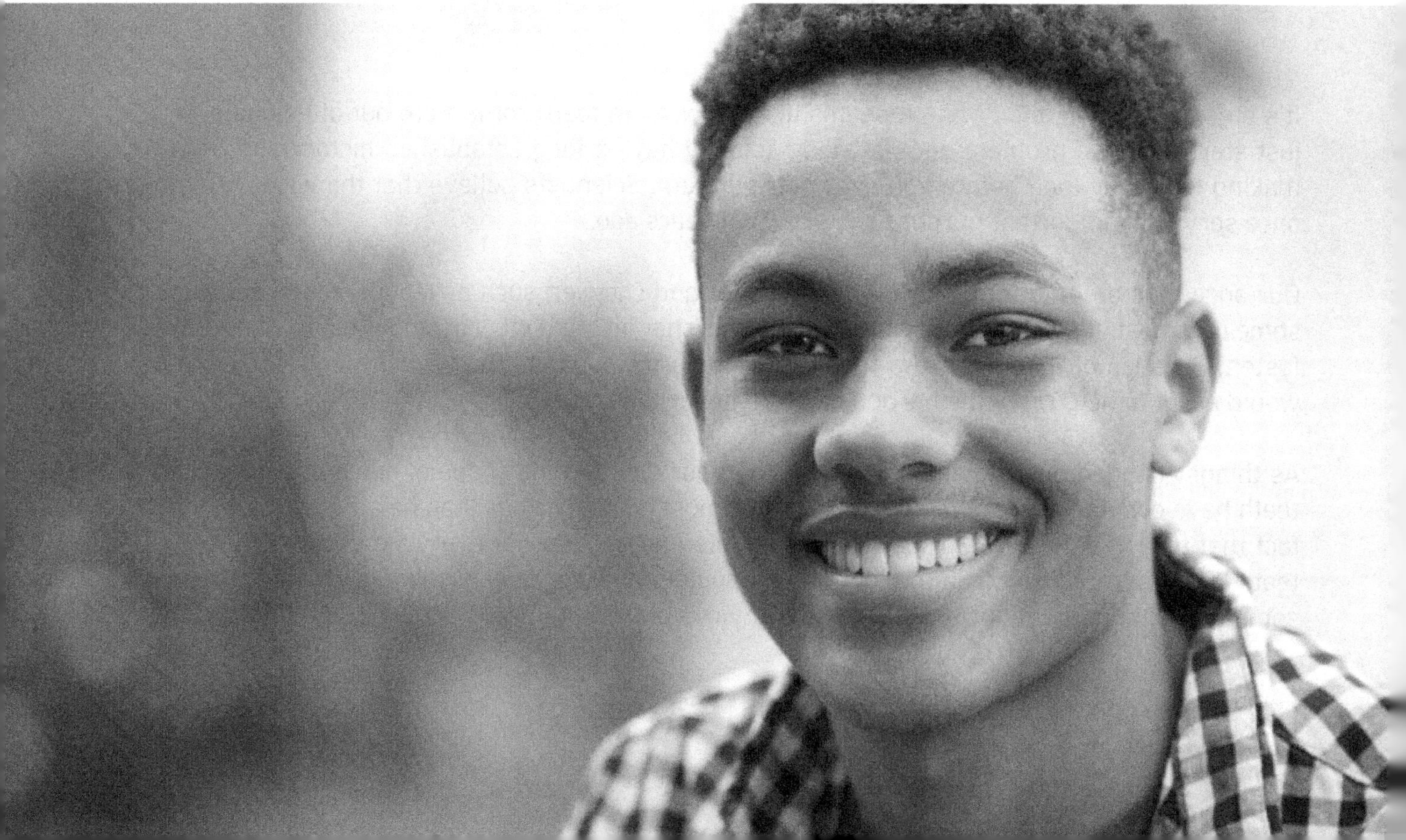

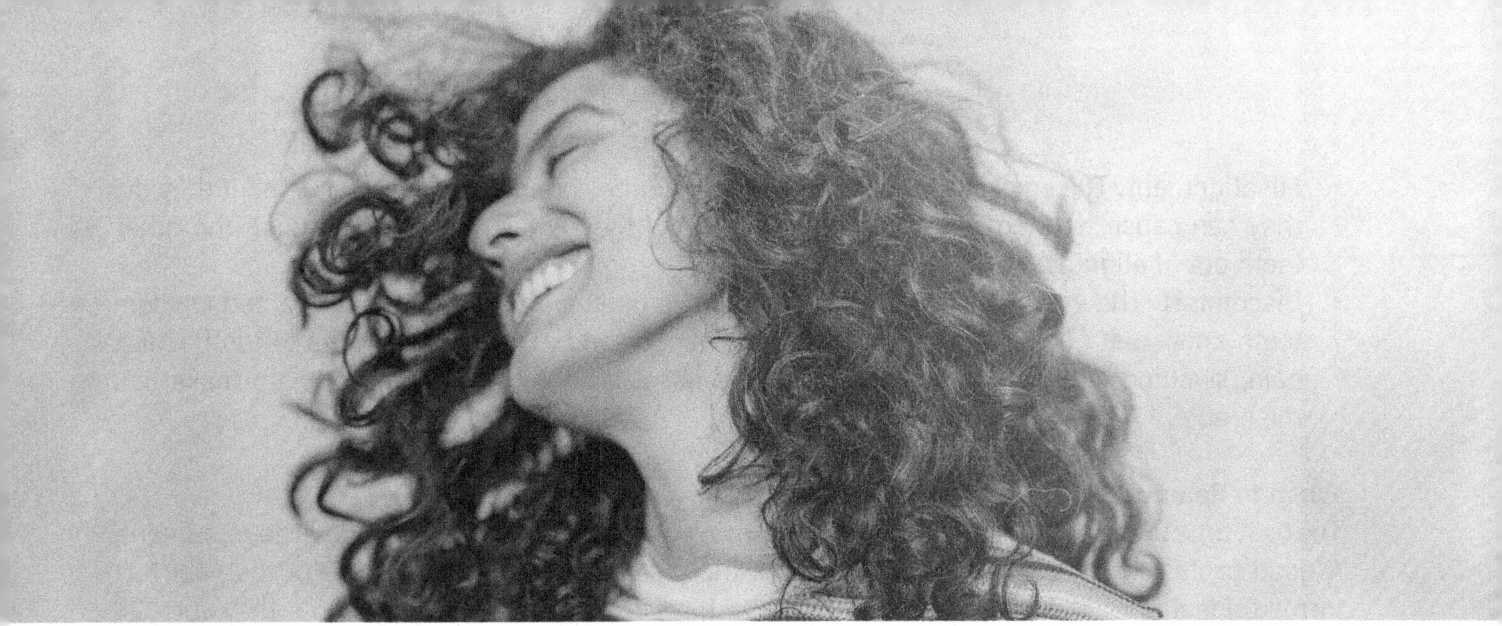

What They Are, Why Removed

Wisdom teeth, also referred to as your third molars, are the larger teeth at the very back of the mouth. They are the last teeth to come in, usually somewhere between the ages of 15 and 25, which is considered to be the "age of wisdom," hence their name. While some people have no problems with their wisdom teeth erupting, many others find that they present a challenge and can be risky to the health of your other teeth.

About the time that this third set of molars begins erupting, some common problems also emerge as a result. Some of the problems associated with erupting wisdom teeth include:

- **Impaction.** According to the National Institutes of Health, wisdom teeth are the most common teeth to become impacted. When a tooth is impacted, it means that the tooth has failed to emerge through the surface of the gum or that only a portion of it has emerged.
- **Caries.** An impacted third molar leads to a high probability of creating dental caries, or cavities, both in that tooth and in the one next to it, as well. This is because they often trap plaque in the area, which is difficult to reach and to clean.
- **Cysts.** When wisdom teeth are impacted, it can cause cysts and tumors to form around the area. This can lead to additional problems because it can affect the bone, and even damage the jaw. Risks with this involve infections, as well as tooth abscesses.

- **Misalignment.** The emerging wisdom teeth may not be coming in straight or, even if they do, they can cause problems with the other teeth. As they emerge, they often push the other teeth out of alignment.
- **Discomfort.** The vast majority of people who have dealt with emerging or impacted wisdom teeth know just how uncomfortable the experience can be. From headaches to toothaches, pain, swelling, and feeling ill, the discomfort associated with wisdom teeth can make you miserable.

When to Remove

The best time to have your third set of molars removed really depends on the tooth's development. A good professional rule of thumb is to have them removed when two-thirds of the root has formed. Ideally, it is recommended that people have them removed by the time they turn 24 years old. This is because it will help to prevent all of the problems listed above and because the ability to re-grow bone in that area of the jaw is reduced as time goes on. Also, the third set of molars is usually easier to remove when you are younger, and the recovery period is also shorter during that time.

The presence of your third set of molars is usually associated with an increased risk of periodontitis, which is an inflammation of the gums and bone, which can lead to tooth loss, abscesses, infections, and tooth shifting. It is important to note, as well, that an absence of symptoms does not mean that there is no problem or disease.

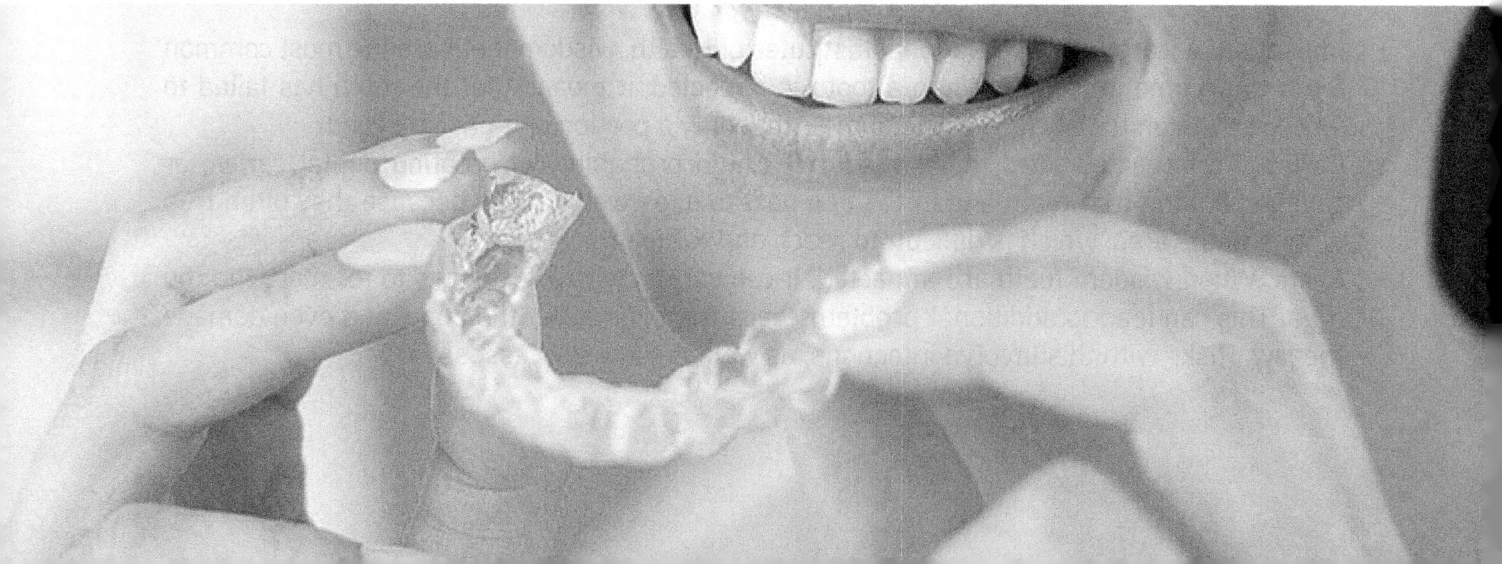

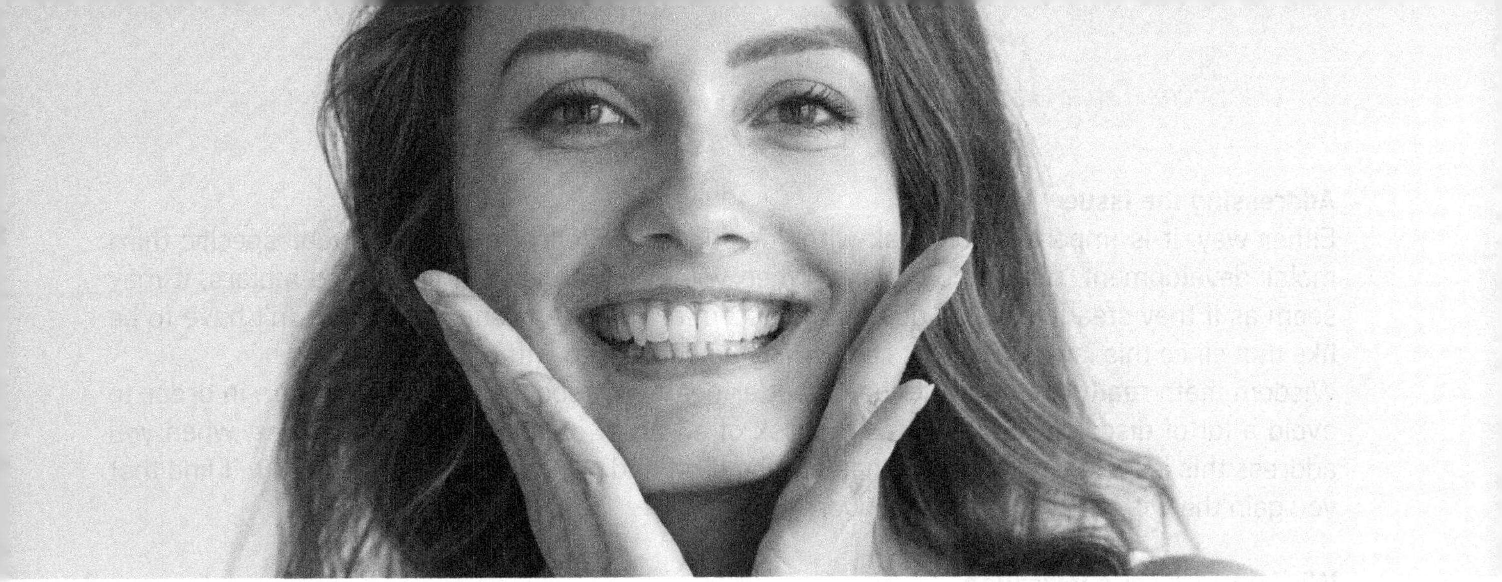

Additionally, research regarding people who did not have their wisdom teeth removed demonstrates that the older they got, the more common it was for them to have cavities in those teeth, as well as in the adjacent ones, due to the difficulties of keeping them properly cleaned. In fact, a 2011 study published in the Journal of Oral and Maxillofacial Surgery reported that, of the nearly 7,000 older adults they studied who had at least one third molar, most of those people had tooth decay or periodontal pathology involving those teeth, and that few had visible molars that were free of disease.

Additional Concerns

There is some controversy regarding whether those who wear a retainer or have had braces in the past need to continue wearing their retainer once the wisdom teeth have been removed. Because there is a risk of relapse if the retainer is not worn, it is recommended that patients continue wearing theirs, as recommended by their orthodontist. Doing so will help to eliminate the risks associated with shifting teeth.

If you are experiencing the emergence of your wisdom teeth, or someone in your family is, be sure you know the facts, risks, and options that are currently available. Having wisdom teeth removed is a common procedure today, and one that most people recover from without issue. Removing third molars can be an important step to take if you are having problems now, or as a preventative measure to avoid issues that can arise later.

Addressing the Issue

Either way, it is important to speak with your doctor to learn more about your specific third molar development, risks, and options. When you are dealing with your third molars, it may seem as if they steal the show, due to the discomfort they can cause. But it doesn't have to be like that since this is an issue that can usually be addressed without difficulty.

Wisdom teeth really are an issue that is better dealt with sooner, rather than later, in order to avoid a lot of discomfort, as well as the risk of an array of complications. Besides, when you address this issue head on, rather than putting it off and prolonging the issue, you will find that you gain the wisdom, without all the worry!

Wisdom Teeth and Invisalign

Understandably, many people are curious about how wisdom teeth and Invisalign fair. Some people who seek Invisalign have not yet had their third molars erupt, while others have had them extracted already, and still others may have wisdom teeth that are partially erupted.

The good news is that no matter what stage your wisdom teeth growth is in, you can still begin the Invisalign treatment program. If you have been working with your dentist about your wisdom teeth, continue to do so in order to address the issue. If the issue of your wisdom teeth arises with the orthodontist, then he or she will explain the best course of action for you to take.

It is also usually acceptable to get wisdom teeth extracted during the Invisalign treatment process. This, of course, is up to the discretion of the orthodontist you are working with, but in most cases it is acceptable. Your Invisalign aligners will be fabricated to account for wisdom teeth that are erupting and getting them extracted during the treatment process should not impede the outcome of the treatment at all.

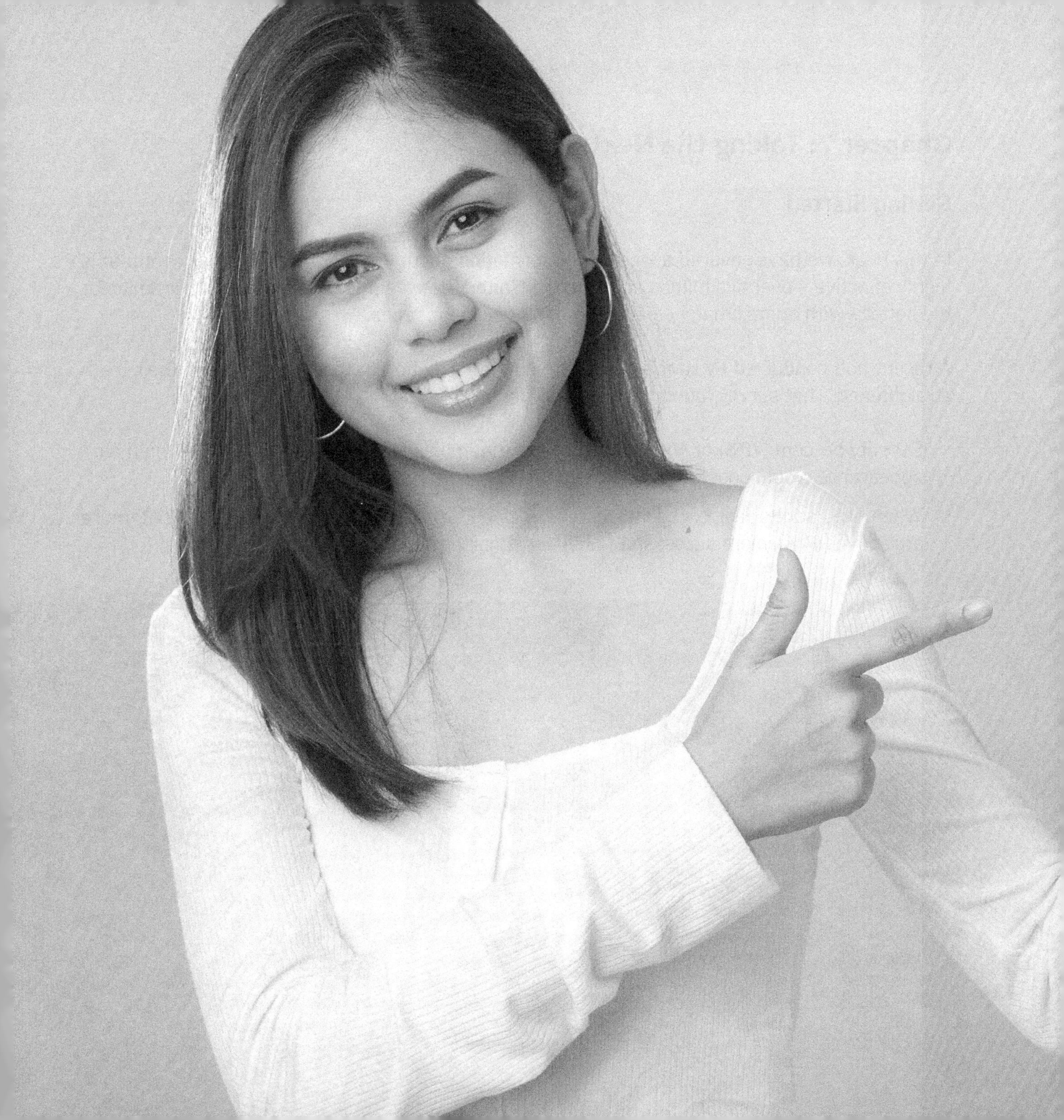

Chapter 7: Taking the Next Step

Getting Started

In this book, we have covered a wealth of information about Invisalign. It is a treatment that is highly effective – over five million adults in the United States alone have changed their smile for the better - with approximately one million of those being teens.

A recent poll conducted by Harris gathered some information from adults who had their teeth straightened. That survey found the following data:

- Seventy percent (70%) of American's believe that making one simple improvement in their appearance would boost their confidence.
- When U.S. adults feel confident, many say people perceive them as happier (63%), more attractive (44%), more successful (43%) and smarter (40%).

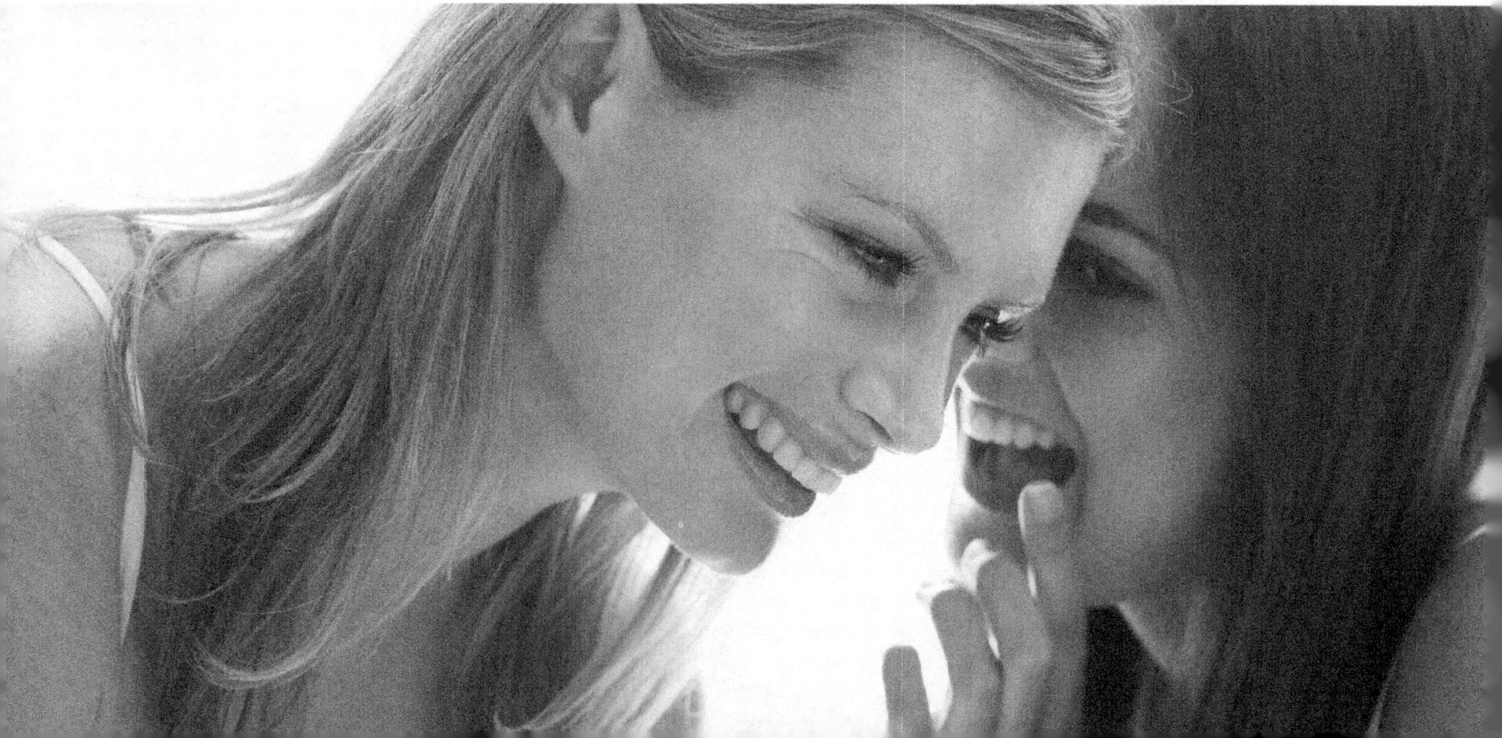

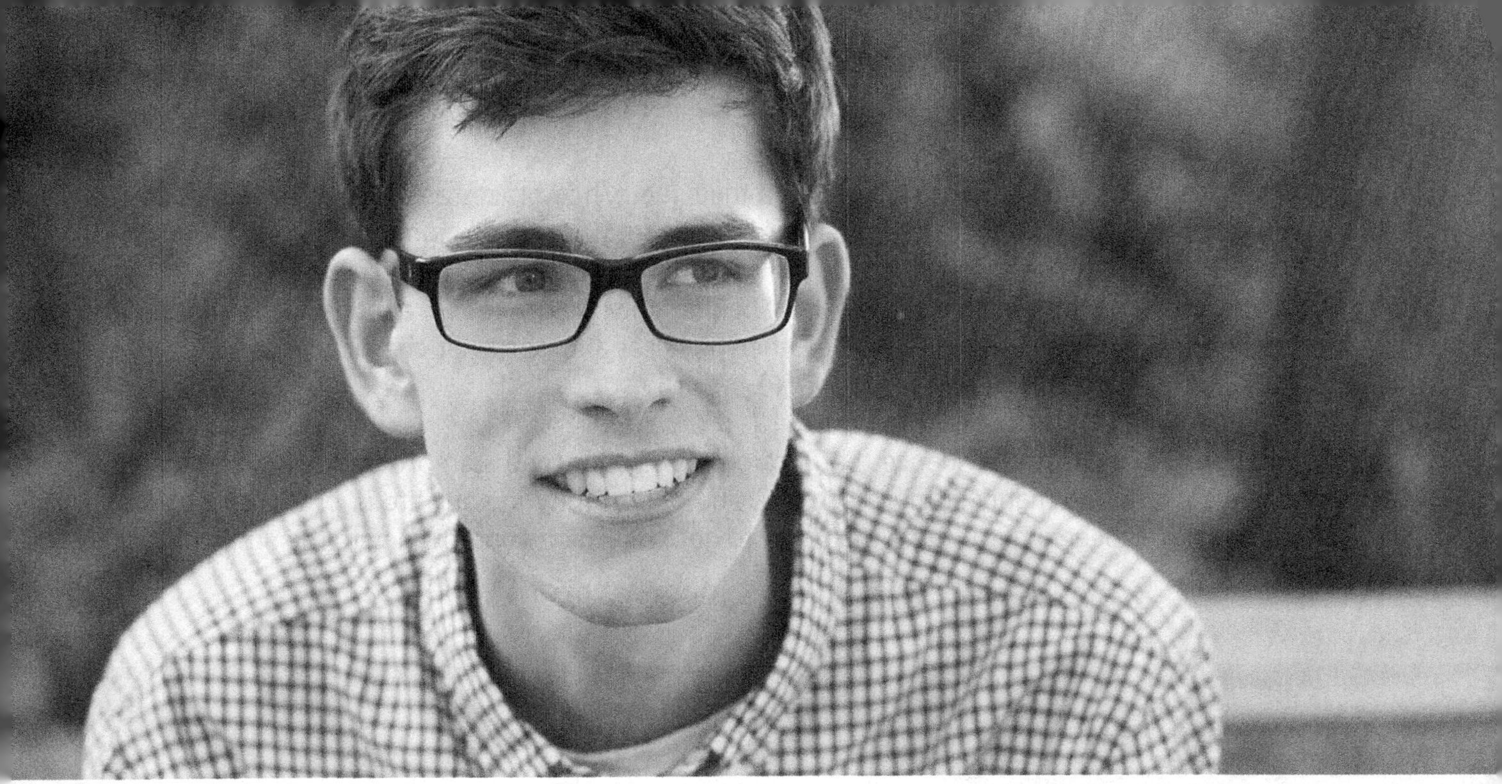

- The desire to have more confidence (38%) and maintaining their health (66%) motivates U.S. adults to make an improvement to their physical appearance.
- Ninety two percent (92%) of adults who have straightened their teeth cite that having straight teeth was important to their confidence.
- Nearly 8 in 10 adults (78%) agree teeth straightening is one of the most important treatments they have ever done for themselves.
- Nearly 8 in 10 adults (78%) agree teeth straightening and has given them the confidence to do something they never could have done before they fixed their teeth.
- Almost 3 in 10 (29%) credit teeth straightening with allowing them to conquer a personal goal.

- Three-quarters of those who straightened their teeth/had braces as an adult experienced at least some positive impact (75%) on their life due to the teeth straightening.

- Today, one's teeth (57%) are the #2 trait, behind only weight (60%), about which Americans continue to feel insecure, surpassing other physical and personal characteristics like nose (50%), personality (35%) and height (27%).

As you can see above, the evidence that straightening your teeth can provide you with the self confidence needed to manifest more success and opportunity in your life is pretty conclusive. There has never been a better time than now to get started on your journey to the smile of your dreams!

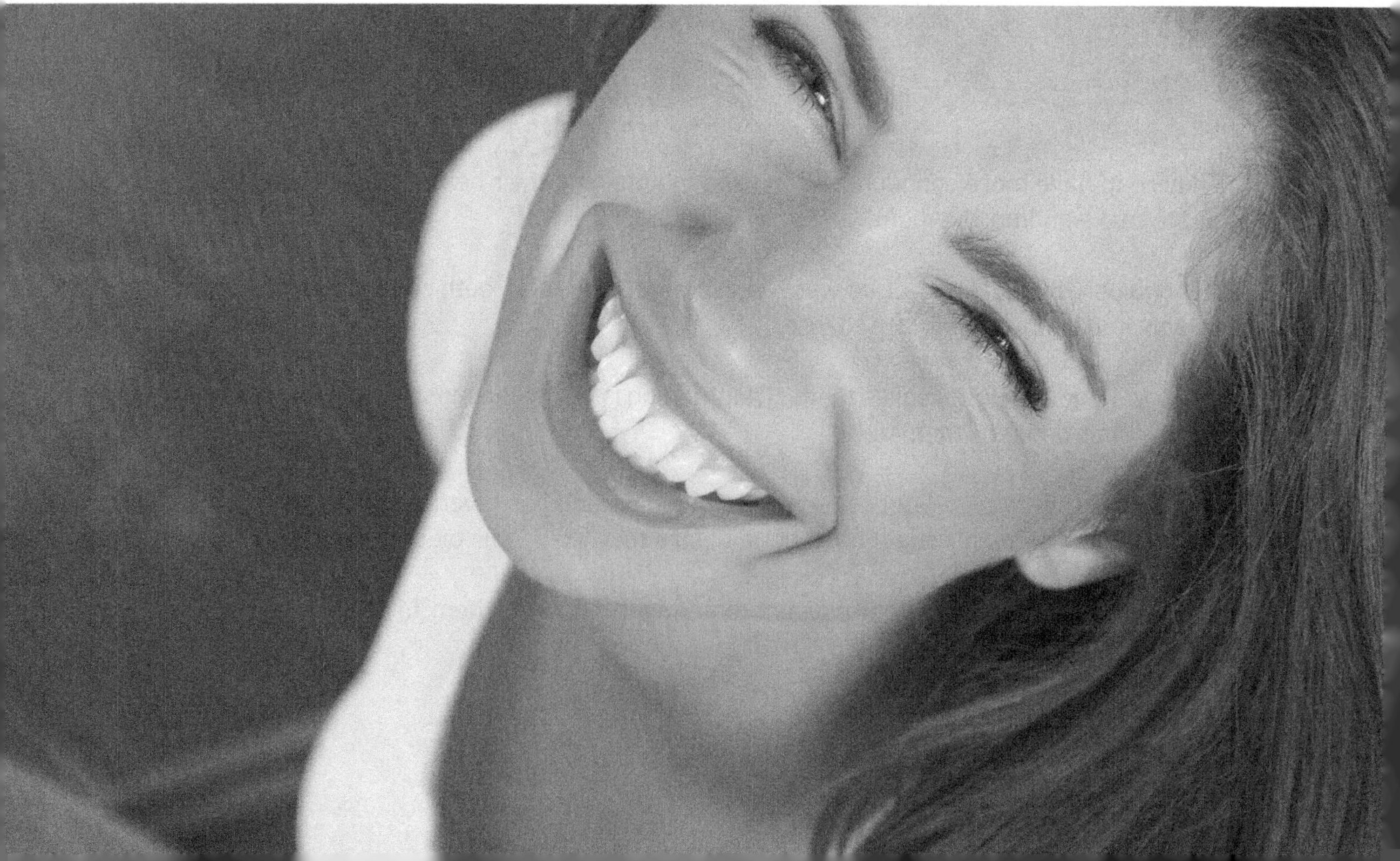

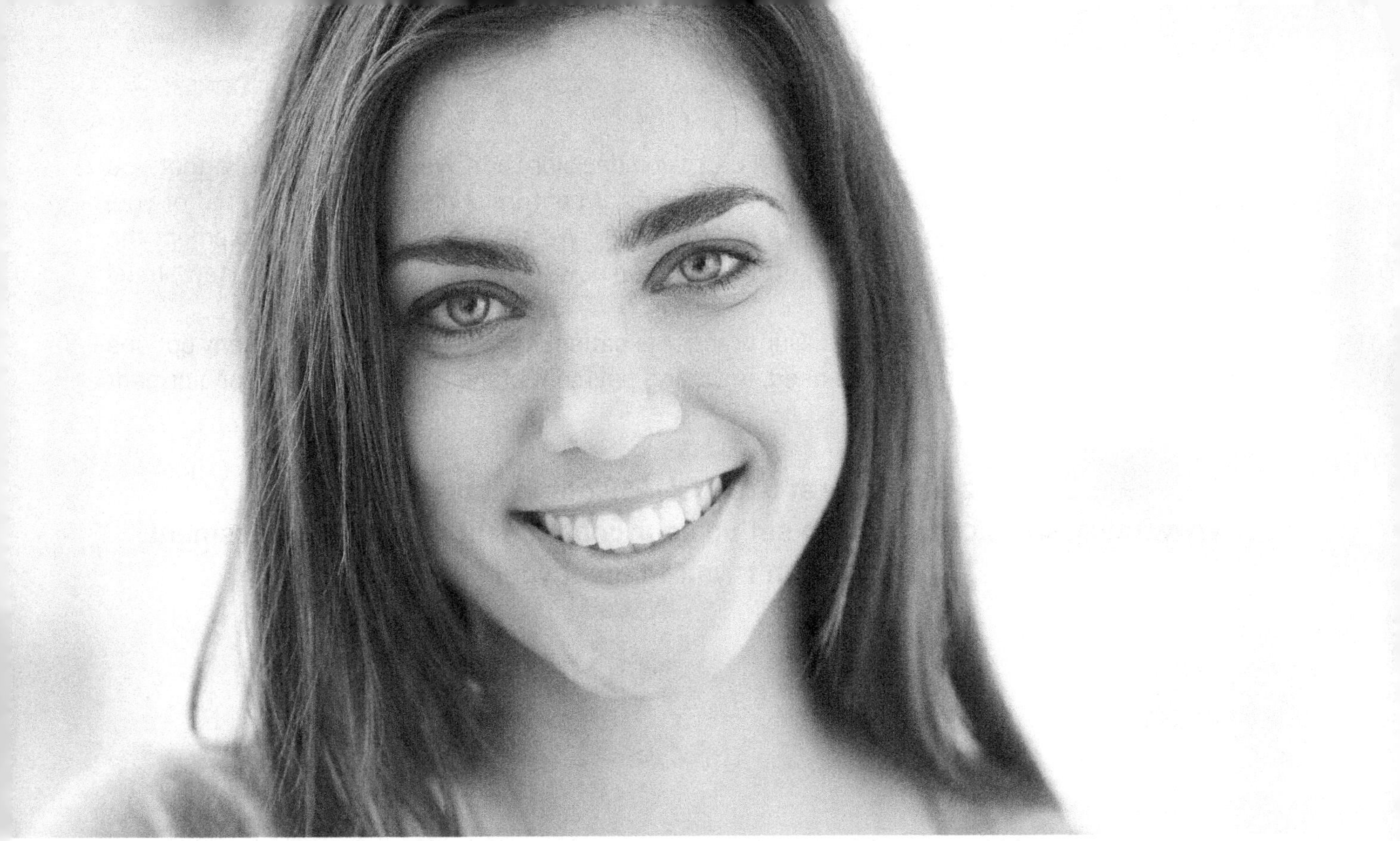

Your Personal Smile Assessment

If you are still unsure if Invisalign is right for you, or you have questions about certain aspects of treatment, addressing your concerns is a phone call or click away. Our friendly and knowledgeable staff can provide you with the answers you need, or can set up an appointment to meet with the doctor and go over your treatment options.

One thing that we advise our patients which we feel is very important: do not be afraid to ask questions. It it recommended that you keep a list of concerns handy while you are doing research or engaging in the decision making process. (We have provided a convenient place in the back of this book to take notes as well).

Having a treatment like Invisalign done is a major decision, and we want to be sure that you are comfortable and aware of exactly what your treatment involves, what is expected of you, and what the process is going to be like start to finish. We are here not only to implement the procedure, but to provide you with expert guidance on how to get the most out of your new smile!

We are a certified Invisalign provider. Our practice is patient focused and offers you many options to be able to get the treatment you need, including payment plans and convenient appointment times.

Give us a call today at 828-254-4602 or visit our website at www.mytsosmile.com today to set up your complimentary smile assessment. We can't wait to meet you!

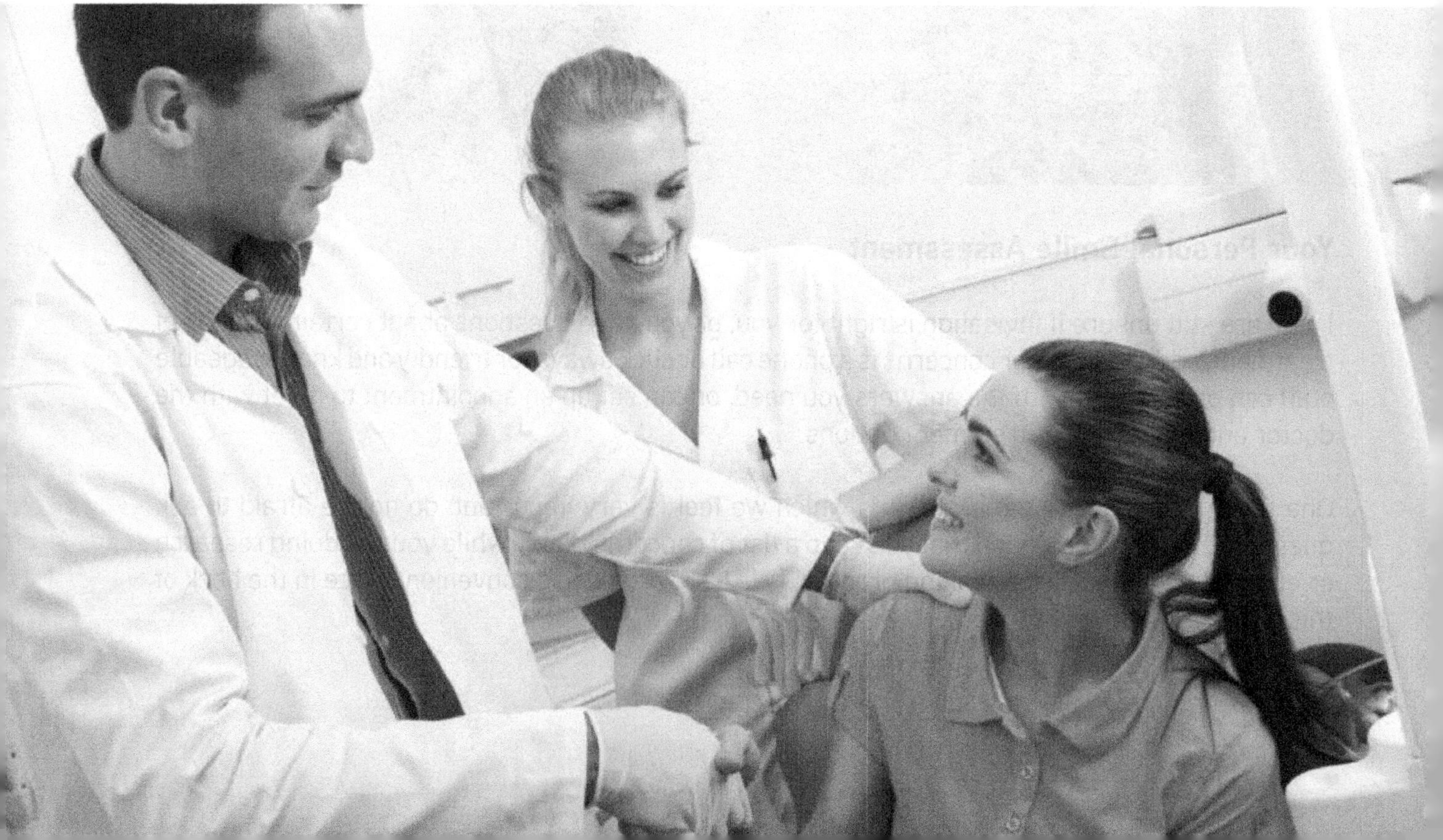

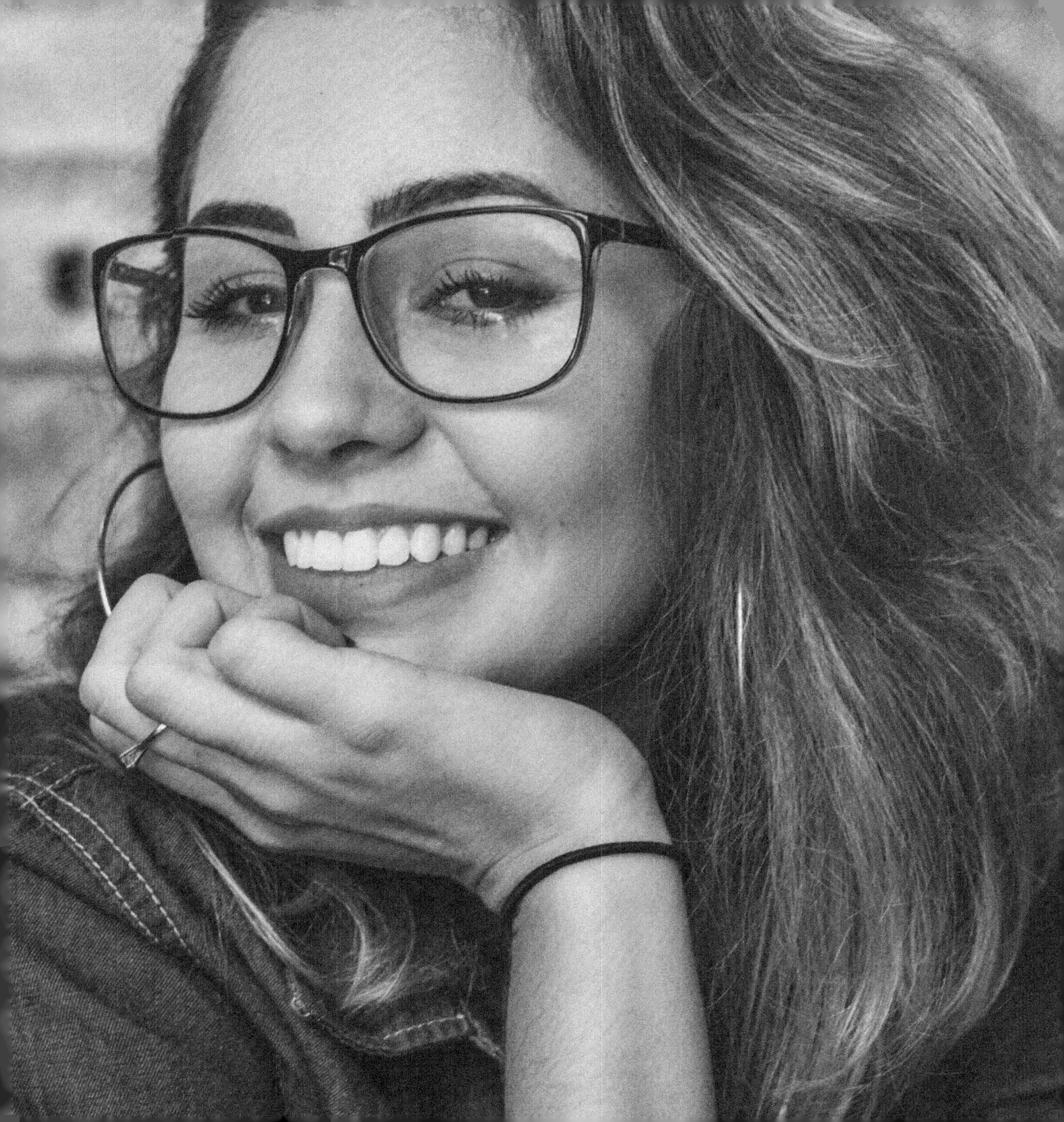

NOTES

NOTES

NOTES

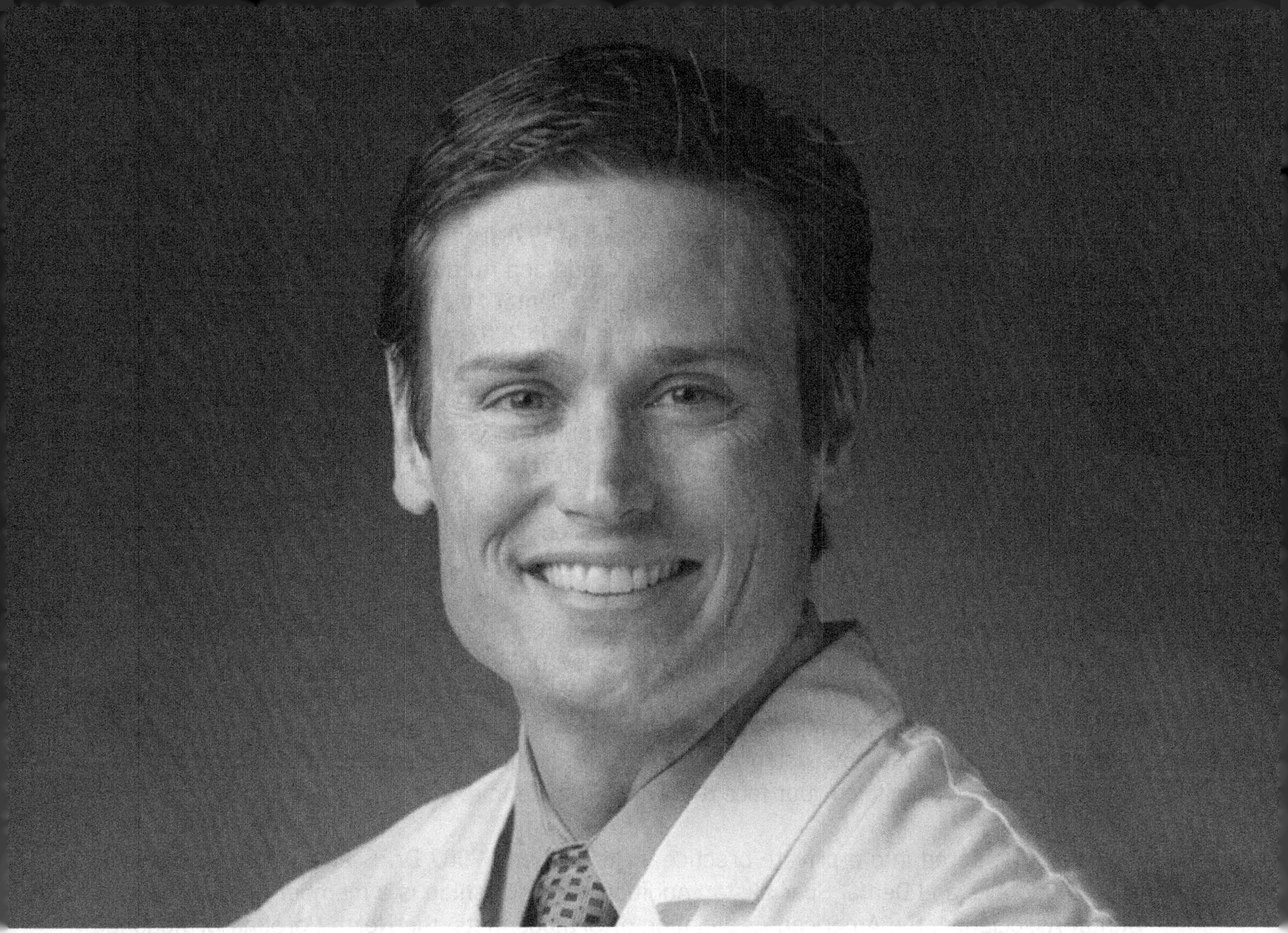

ABOUT THE AUTHOR

When you meet Dr. Scanlan you will find him to be a warm compassionate person that always puts the needs of his patients first. He puts a high value on both your concerns and those of your children. Having you and your child enjoy and understand the steps along the way and have a clear vision of what's at the end of the orthodontic journey is the goal of Dr. Scanlan and his team.

Here is a little bit about Dr. Scanlan's journey.

Dr. Scanlan received his Bachelor of Science degree in 1998 from the University of North Carolina at Charlotte, where he graduated Magna Cum Laude and number one in his class. Following college, Dr. Scanlan was accepted at the School of Dental Medicine at the State University of New York at Buffalo. There, he graduated Cum Laude in 2002.

Upon graduation from dental school, Dr. Scanlan was commissioned into the United States Army as a captain assigned to the Dental Corps. During his first year in the Army, he completed the one-year Advance General Dentistry program from the United States Army Medical Department at Fort Benning, Georgia. Upon completion of this additional training, he began a three-year assignment at Fort Sill, Oklahoma, where he practiced general dentistry and operated his own clinic.

During his training and service in the Army, Dr. Scanlan solidified his desire to make a difference in other's lives through their smiles. This desire led Dr. Scanlan to career in orthodontics. He completed a three-year post-doctoral Master's degree and certification in orthodontics in 2009 at the Mayo Clinic in Rochester, Minnesota. At the Mayo Clinic, he received state-of-the-art training in orthodontics that will move you or your child quickly through the orthodontic experience to a result that leaves a smile on your face that will last a lifetime.

Dr. Scanlan entered into a private practice in Asheville in 2009 Dr. Scanlan is the founder of TS Orthodontics and Dental Specialists. Additionally, Dr Scanlan is a member of the American Dental Association, the American Association of Orthodontists, the North Carolina Orthodontic Association and the Southern Association of Orthodontists.

Dr. Scanlan is married to Amy Scanlan of Concord, North Carolina. They met in college at the University of North Carolina at Charlotte. They have two children - Hunter and Emma who are enjoying the great life that Asheville offers a family.

When you meet Dr. Scanlan and his team you will immediately get a sense of his devotion to making smiles and contributing to his community.

Made in the USA
Monee, IL
08 November 2026

67380764R00083